Everyday Pediatrics for Parents and Caretakers

The ABCs of Common Problems in Child Health

George Salamon M.D. FAAP.

PAGE PUBLISHING
Conneaut Lake, PA

First originally published by Page Publishing 2024

ISBN 979-8-88654-224-0 (pbk)
ISBN 979-8-88654-237-0 (digital)

Printed in the United States of America

I dedicate this book to all the parents who trusted me with the medical care of their children throughout the decades.

Contents

Acknowledgments

I am indebted to Professor Phillip Brunell for being my mentor, reviewing my manuscript, and giving me many advices.

I appreciate Professor Martha Satz for editing my manuscript and giving me advice.

I am thankful to Mr. Peter Dressner for helping me with all the computer work necessary for my book.

I want to thank Page Publishing for publishing my book and to every person there who was involved with my book.

I am grateful to my wife, Eva, for managing my pediatric office and giving me advice through the decades, making it possible for me to concentrate exclusively on patient care.

Introduction

I am George Salamon, MD, FAAP, a board-certified pediatrician who has worked in pediatrics for fifty years. In addition, I was a clinical assistant professor at Southwestern Medical School Department of Pediatrics and chief of pediatrics at Medical Center Plano (present name Medical City Plano). I have been affiliated with six hospitals, including Children's Medical Center Dallas.

In this book, I want to share with you my knowledge and experience. My goal is to bring everyday pediatrics closer to you, the parents and caretakers. I think I know what parents do not know in general and they would need to, what advices they can use, and learn the common misconceptions.

I have not intended to talk about every aspect of pediatrics but about common problems and important issues.

I have also included routine baby care.

I have emphasized the important points by repeating them throughout the text. I also have repetitions in order to avoid the need for you to go back to different chapters all the time. Although I mentioned those chapters if you want to go back. They are in parentheses.

I have written in the style I use to speak with patients and their parents.

After the chapter general and safety advices, I tried to organize chapters of the book in alphabetical order.

When your child needs medical attention, I referred to *the* doctor instead of *a* doctor, because your child gets the best care if he goes to the doctor who regularly sees him, knows his medical history, and provides him a so-called medical home.

I think my book is unique because of the following:

1. Many chapters start with a list of important questions that pediatricians ask parents. After the parents answer those questions, the doctor has a good medical history, which is half of the diagnosis.
2. Then I start with the symptoms, and I group them, leading to possible diagnoses. This way you can get a glimpse of pediatric diagnosis and decision-making.
   I wanted to show the significant symptoms and diseases that need immediate medical attention.
3. My last chapter lists and explains many tests, procedures, and surgeries. It also describes the work of different health professionals.

The Well Child

A. The unborn child—fetus

The fetus, the baby-to-be, is well protected in the womb (uterus) inside the so-called amniotic sac in the amniotic fluid. The amniotic fluid surrounds and protects the fetus during pregnancy. But some things can harm the fetus. I want you to know about them so you can avoid exposure and protect your baby.

The unborn child is called a fetus from the eighth week after conception until birth. Your obstetrician will monitor the growth and maturity of your fetus and may order an ultrasound or ultrasounds, which uses high-frequency sound waves and produces images of internal organs (see tests, procedures, surgeries). Ultrasonography is used routinely today during pregnancy to see how the fetus is developing and to determine if the baby is having any problems. Ultrasonography is a safe tool to use because there is no radiation like there is with an x-ray. If there is any suspicion of a genetic problem like Down syndrome, an amniocentesis can be performed (see tests, procedures, surgeries).

The well-being of the fetus is regularly checked. To feel the movements of the fetus and hear the heart sounds are important.

How old the fetus is—called the gestational age—is determined by dating the mother's last menstrual period. A full-term pregnancy is forty weeks. It is very important that a woman live the best healthy life she can during these forty weeks—everything she does can affect the baby. A healthy lifestyle and good nutrition help the growth and development of the fetus.

Agents and infections that can harm the fetus.

Different *agents and infections* can hurt the baby while in utero—developing inside the womb.

The fetus is most vulnerable in the first twelve weeks of life.

Many drugs that are safe for women when they are not pregnant can affect the developing fetus; therefore, it is important for a pregnant woman to check with her doctor about what medicines she can safely take.

Alcohol, illicit drugs, and tobacco in all forms can also cause fetal harm. It is imperative that mothers refrain from drinking and taking drugs and quit smoking to give their child the best chances to develop into a healthy baby.

Viruses, bacteria, and parasites can also harm the developing fetus, so talk with your doctor if you are sick.

Agents that can harm the fetus: alcohol, drug use disorder, and tobacco use of the mother

Alcohol

If the mother is a chronic drinker of alcohol, the baby can be born with a condition called "fetal alcohol syndrome," which is a group of conditions that include physical and mental problems that can affect the child's behavior and learning. The alcohol in the blood passes to the baby through the umbilical cord. No amount of alcohol is safe for the fetus.

In many areas, the baby may be affected if born with *fetal alcohol syndrome*. The baby's height and weight can be less than other babies, which is called small for gestational age (SGA), and the child might have a condition called failure to thrive (FTT). That means that the weight is lagging behind. (See failure to thrive.)

The infant can be born with a small head called microcephaly (see large, small, and misshapen head). Intellectual disability of some degree is often present.

There are characteristic features of the face, affecting the look of the eyes, nose, and mouth. The philtrum (an indentation above the upper lip) is absent.

Drugs

Opioids, which are used to manage pain are highly addictive and are one of the most common drugs that are misused. They can cause serious problems for the developing fetus, including preterm birth, still birth, and birth defects. Even a baby who makes it to term—the full forty weeks—is likely to have problems. A newborn born to a woman who is a drug abuser may suffer from withdrawal symptoms after birth that can start on the first day of life or a few days later. They will suffer irritability, excessive crying, and tremor. Excessive sweating, vomiting, diarrhea, and seizures can occur too.

These newborns need to be undisturbed, kept in a quiet, somewhat dark area in the nursery. They may also be given medications if the symptoms are really bad.

The mother should be treated for drug use disorder. But women who remain drug-free can breastfeed. Her physician may regularly test the urine to make sure that she is drug-free.

No marijuana or any kind of drug should be used by a mother during pregnancy and breastfeeding unless prescribed by her doctor.

Tobacco

Tobacco use during pregnancy can result in many problems for the unborn child. Tobacco can cause the baby to be born early, have low birth weight, and birth defects. Smoking can damage a baby's lungs. Tobacco use also increases the risk for sudden infant death syndrome. Secondhand smoke is not harmless either.

E-cigarettes and other tobacco products contain nicotine, and chemicals are also harmful during pregnancy.

Infections that can harm the fetus

Viruses: rubella, cytomegalovirus, herpesvirus, chicken pox, human immunodeficiency virus (HIV), Zika virus.
Bacteria: syphilis
Parasite: toxoplasma

Congenital rubella

It is a viral infection.
The fetus gets infected during the first trimester. After birth, sputum can be the source of infection.
Symptoms are severe vision and hearing problems, mental retardation, heart disease.
No treatment is available.
Prevention is very important with vaccination prior to pregnancy (MMR vaccine).
(See rubella.)

Cytomegalovirus

It is a viral infection that can cause severe congenital disease.
The newborn can get infected by secretion containing the virus, through the placenta, the infected birth canal, and breast milk.
Most babies have no symptoms at birth.
Symptoms are jaundice that develops shortly after birth. The liver and spleen get enlarged. Rash- blood spots (purpura) develop. Severe vision and hearing problems, mental retardation, and microcephaly (very small head) can be consequences of the infection.
Treatment for symptomatic neonates is Valganciclovir by mouth for six months.
Antiviral medications are somewhat effective.
Prevention: good handwashing, particularly after diaper change.

Herpesvirus

Herpesvirus type 1 (HSV-1) primarily causes gingivostomatitis (swelling and redness of the gums and blisters). It may affect the thumb in thumb-suckers.
Herpesvirus type 2 (HSV-2) involves the genitalia.
The newborn can be infected during vaginal delivery of a mother who is infected.
Herpes can affect different organs, causing severe diseases.
Inflammation of the brain (encephalitis) is the most severe.
Diagnosis is made by tests from the blisters.
Treatment is antiviral medications, like acyclovir.

Chicken pox

It is a viral disease.
Congenital chicken pox (varicella) occurs when the fetus is exposed to chicken pox infection early in pregnancy. The risk is highest when the mother is infected during thirteen to twenty weeks of gestation.
When a pregnant woman develops chicken pox around the time of the delivery, the neonate can get sick.
Infants whose mother develops chicken pox five days before or two days after delivery are at risk for severe disease.
These babies should be treated with varicella-zoster immune globulin. Antiviral medication is also available.
Prevention is very important with immunization (chicken pox vaccine called Varivax or a combination of measles, mumps, rubella, and chicken pox vaccines called ProQuad or MMRV). However, pregnant women should not get these vaccines.

Human immunodeficiency virus (HIV)

The newborn can get this virus from the mother through the placenta, during birth, and from breast milk.

The infants have low birth weight and failure to thrive (FTT) (see failure to thrive).

Lymph nodes, the liver, and spleen can be enlarged.

Continuous thrush in the mouth (candidiasis) is suspicious of an immune problem, including HIV.

Chronic diarrhea and pneumonia are common.

Chronic and recurrent bacterial and viral infections are frequent. The bacterial infection includes tuberculosis (TB).

The diagnosis is made by laboratory tests.

Antiviral drugs are available to treat mother and child.

Zika virus

This virus is transmitted to people through the bite of infected mosquitoes and sexual contact.

The virus is mostly present in Central and South America, the Caribbean, but a few cases have occurred in South Florida and Texas.

The mother can have mild symptoms or no symptoms at all but still can pass the virus to the fetus.

Symptoms are fever, rash, pink eye, joint pain.

The newborn can be born with birth defects, small head (microcephaly) (see large, small and misshapen head) and consequent mental retardation.

The diagnosis is made by laboratory tests.

No treatment or vaccine is available.

Prevention: Pregnant women and women planning to get pregnant should try to avoid areas where Zika virus is prevalent. They need to protect themselves from mosquito bites (net, spray), and during sex.

Congenital syphilis

It is caused by a bacteria called Treponema pallidum, and it is a sexually transmitted disease (STD).

The germ is transmitted to the newborn by the placenta.

Some infected children have no symptoms at birth.

Symptoms are rash, enlarged liver and spleen, jaundice. Bone disease can occur, and infection of the membrane around the brain (meningitis) is not uncommon.

Blood tests are available to make the diagnosis and screen pregnant women.

Treatment is antibiotics for both mother and baby.

(See sexually transmitted diseases.)

Toxoplasmosis

Toxoplasma is a single cell parasite.

Cats can transmit the disease. They often hunt infected rodents.

Uncooked or undercooked meat, soil, and untreated water also can be contaminated with toxoplasma.

Infants with congenital infections can be symptom-free at birth.

However, the baby can have severe visual impairment, hearing loss, learning disabilities, mental retardation that can show up months or even years later.

Calcification in the brain and increased amount of fluid in the chambers (ventricles) of the brain (hydrocephalus) (see large, small, and misshapen head) are characteristic of congenital toxoplasma infection.

The diagnosis is made by laboratory tests.

Treatment: medications.

Prevention is important. The tools are good handwashing, cooking or baking the meat thoroughly (dried and smoked meat are not safe). Wash and rub the fruits and vegetables several times. Avoid drinking untreated water and raw milk. Pregnant women should not change the cat litter.

B. *The newborn infant*

After birth

After birth, the newborn is placed on a radiant warmer. Once suction of secretions and drying are complete, the condition of the newborn is evaluated. Often the so-called *Apgar score* is used. The heart rate, respiratory effort, muscle tone, color, and response to stimulus are assessed. These signs are checked at one and five minutes after birth. For example, an Apgar score of eight out of ten is a high score. It means that the baby is doing well. After the evaluation, the baby is swaddled. In the nursery, the infant's weight, height, and head size is measured. Following the measurements, the nurse places the baby back on the warmer. The infant's temperature and vital signs are checked, and a physical exam is done. Then the baby receives an eye ointment and vitamin K shot. This shot is very important to prevent bleeding. In a few hours, if the infant's temperature is stable, the baby receives a sponge bath. Lately, skin-to-skin contact is practiced as well until the first breastfeeding is finished. Healthy infants can be placed belly down to the mother's chest. They get dried and covered with a blanket.

The doctor will see the baby and do a physical exam in the first twenty-four hours. Common findings at the first physical exam include the following:

- The head is often elongated after birth.
- Soft swelling or a bump (caput succedaneum) on the head is not uncommon.
- Some babies have cephalhematoma. That is a swelling on the head under the scalp after birth. It is caused by accumulation of blood from pressure and located on one side of the head.
- The baby's eyelids can be swollen.
- Red bloody spots may appear in the baby's eyes due to the pressure from going through the birth canal. These spots will resolve over time.
- Swelling of the breasts (mastitis neonatorum) is not uncommon.

- Boys sometimes have swelling on one or both testicles that usually resolves by one year of age (*hydrocele*).

Hypospadias. This is a birth defect. The opening of the penis where the urine passes is on the underside instead of the tip of the penis where it normally is. Also, some foreskin is missing. The circumcision needs to wait because the treatment is surgery, and the foreskin is used. The condition is usually noted in the nursery with the physical exam. Consultation with a urologist is necessary.

If your son is to be *circumcised*, that is done in the treatment room of the nursery. Do not get the area of the circumcision wet. Petroleum jelly and a loose sterile gauze is used over the penis. If there is any redness, swelling, yellow or green discharge, call the doctor. Circumcision usually heals within a week.

Girls may have white mucus or blood in the vaginal area, caused by maternal hormones.

The skin of the newborn is usually red, and birthmarks are common. Birthmarks include red spots, "stork bites," and bluish bruise-like marks called Mongolian spots. These birthmarks do not cause any problems (see birthmarks).

Newborn babies sometimes breathe differently than older children. Their breathing can slow down and even stop for a few seconds before rapidly coming back. This is called periodic breathing. If there is no color change and if the incident does not last longer than twenty seconds, it is normal. However, if the lips or face turn blue or purple, that is abnormal, and emergency care is needed. A nurse should be called into the hospital room right away.

Sneezing, sniffling, and hiccups are all normal.

Newborn babies often have rashes (newborn acne, milia, pustular melanosis, erythema toxicum) (see below).

Newborn acne (acne neonatorum). They are small bumps on the face, nose, forehead, but often on the trunk too. The acne usually disappears without treatment.

Milia. These are small white bumps not requiring treatment because it resolves.

Pustular melanosis. This is a condition with small bumps and brownish spots anywhere on the skin. It resolves by itself.

Erythema toxicum. Small red areas on the skin with small white bumps. It has a spontaneous resolution.

Torticollis. Newborns can have torticollis, when the baby's head is tilted and he has problems turning it. A small lump often can be palpated on the side of the neck. It resolves after a while, and physiotherapy can be helpful.

Fracture of the collarbone can occur. (See broken bones.)

Before your baby leaves the newborn nursery, a newborn screening test is done. A blood sample is drawn and sent to the state lab to screen for some diseases. The test needs to be repeated at two weeks of age. This test screens for rare but very serious diseases.

A hearing test is done as well. If it does not give evidence of the infant's normal hearing, the test needs to be repeated.

Another screening is conducted before the newborn leaves the hospital. That looks for any congenital heart disease that did not show clinical signs. The oxygenation of the baby's blood is checked with a routine pulse oximeter screening.

Premature babies undergo a predischarge "car seat challenge." They are seated in the car seat, and their heart rate, breathing, and oxygenation are monitored.

Be sure that in the first few weeks after delivery, you do not touch plants with soil. If the navel gets dirty with soil, the baby can get *tetanus* (*neonatal tetanus*) with devastating consequences. It also can hurt you.

Preparing to take your baby home

During your pregnancy, you probably brought everything the baby will need when arriving home.

The crib, the mattress, changing table, clothes, pajamas, blankets, diapers, wipes, diaper creams, washcloth, towels, bottles, pacifiers.

Buy clothes a little larger than your baby's age because he will grow out of his clothes quickly.

Be sure that everything you buy is up to standard, and safety is your number one priority.

At home with your newborn baby

First of all, keep the baby warm. The room temperature is right when the baby is content. The baby should not be sweating, and the hands and feet should not be cold and purple. It is important to keep the baby on his or her back, not on the tummy or side to prevent sudden infant death syndrome. The baby needs to sleep on a firm mattress (see sudden infant death syndrome [SIDS]).

Keep soft objects, pillows, stuffed animals, and soft bedding out of the crib to prevent suffocation. The baby needs to sleep in the parents' room at least in the first six months but preferably one year. That way you can observe him or her all the time. Do not sleep in the same bed with your baby, because you can injure him or her. Do not swaddle for sleep so he or she can freely move and kick, helping the hips to develop.

To have a baby is a wonderful thing, but it is very demanding, particularly in the first few weeks. If you feel overwhelmed, sad, and hopeless all the time, let your doctor know. These symptoms can be secondary to postpartum depression. During the first few weeks, babies need to eat regularly, which means you need to wake up your baby for feedings. Breastfed babies need to eat every two or two and a half hours. Formula-fed babies need to eat every three hours. After the feeding is well-established and weight gain assured by the pediatrician, you can listen to your baby about when and how much he or she wants to eat. In general, do not feed more than every two hours, and do not wait longer than four hours. After a few months, the majority of babies do not need to eat at night, but premature babies and babies with low birth weight do.

Newborns usually lose weight after birth. But it should be less than 10% of the birth weight. If the newborn lost 10% or more of the birth weight, urgent medical attention is needed. Newborns usually regain their birth weight at two weeks of age and gain about two pounds in the first month.

Babies need to have four to six wet diapers within twenty-four hours and at least one stool every day or every other day.

Both baby girls and boys can have enlarged breasts in the first few weeks, secondary to hormones received from Mom. The navel cord stump (after the umbilical cord is cut at birth, some tissue remains at the baby's belly button, called umbilical cord stump) usually falls off at two to three weeks of age, but this can occur earlier or later. If it is still attached in one month, let the baby's doctor know. You should also alert your doctor if there is discharge from the belly button beyond two weeks of age. It can signal the presence of extra tissue at the umbilicus (*umbilical granuloma*) that the doctor can treat. If there is foul-smelling yellow or green discharge from the navel and/or redness and swelling at the navel cord, that can indicate infection. If that occurs, call the doctor right away. Do not submerge your baby while bathing until the cord stump falls off and the navel is dry and completely healed. Until then, only give your baby sponge baths. When you give a bath, always support the baby's head and neck, and hold the arm so he won't slide. You never can leave your baby or child until eight years of age alone in the bathtub, not even for a second.

If the baby has a temperature of one hundred degrees or more, measured under the arm during the first two to three months, that is an emergency. Go to the emergency room.

Many babies have **colic** with symptoms of fussiness, crying for a long time, and screaming. They often kick or pull their legs up, their face becomes red, and they pass gas. Colic can be very frustrating, even frightening. However, if it is only colic, it is common and not dangerous. Babies usually grow out of colic in two to three months. It is difficult to treat colic, but you can try a few things.

Increase your baby's burping time by placing the baby on your shoulder for thirty to forty-five minutes. You can also hold the baby against your abdomen. A mother who is breastfeeding should keep an eye on her diet. Avoid or limit Coke, coffee, beans, cabbage, broccoli, chocolate, and spicy foods. However, if the baby is inconsolable, vomits, and the abdomen becomes distended, take him or her to the emergency room.

Spitting up is a common problem. It is normal to spit up a small amount of milk, like one teaspoon or a tablespoon. But if it is more significant and affects weight gain, see the doctor. The first remedy for spitting up is also increased burping. Spit-up can be caused by overfeeding, which is a problem that you should discuss with the doctor.

Not all babies have stools every day. Breastfed babies may not have a bowel movement for three days. If there is no stool after three days, call the doctor. On the other end of the spectrum, babies can have three to four bowel movements a day. Breastfed babies may have six to eight yellow stools a day. However, if the baby has frequent stools that contain blood or mucus or have a foul smell, the baby needs to be seen by the doctor. If your baby doesn't urinate for more than eight to nine hours, go to the emergency room.

The urine and stool can cause diaper rash if the diaper is not changed often enough. To avoid diaper rash, apply diaper cream after each diaper change.

Babies can develop jaundice, usually in the first few days after birth. When a baby develops jaundice, his or her skin will turn yellow. The whites of the eyes will also take on a yellow tinge.

Be sure that after leaving the hospital, you make an early appointment with the pediatrician so he or she can notice if jaundice has developed or the baby has any problem. If the baby had jaundice in the hospital, that needs to be monitored.

In most cases, jaundice disappears by the first month of age. But if jaundice persists after a month or it appears later, let the doctor know.

The baby needs another appointment at two weeks of age when the second newborn screening test is done. That is very important.

How do you cut your baby's nails?

Use a pair of blunt baby scissors and be very careful. You can do it when your baby sleeps, but someone needs to hold him and his arm while you cut the nails.

Crying

Babies often cry, particularly at night. They cry when they are hungry or wet. They cry from stomachache, colic, or from pain when they are sick.

You want to pick up your baby and hold him. If he stops crying and smiles, that means he is okay.

But if he continues to cry, you need to check:

- Is he hungry?
- Is his diaper wet?
- Is he warm?
- Are his hands and feet cold?
- Does he act okay?
- Did he vomit or have diarrhea?
- Does his stomach look okay and not distended?

If he feels warm, check his temperature.

Look him over to be sure he does not have a rash, redness, or swelling anywhere, and no hair is caught around his finger.

If he does not stop crying—that is, if he is inconsolable, urgent medical attention is needed.

However, if he vomits and has a swollen abdomen, go to the emergency room, or call 911.

If the baby has a piercing, high-pitched cry, his condition can be secondary to a neurologic condition. In that case, see the doctor or go to the emergency room.

Hiccup

Babies can have hiccups one time or another.

If it occurs when you feed the baby, stop the feeding and burp him. If the hiccup does not stop after a few minutes, you can give him a few sips of sugar water. Put one teaspoon of sugar to four ounces of boiled water. Remember babies cannot have more than one or maximum two ounces of water over twenty-four hours. If he needs more, give Pedialyte.

Jitteriness

Newborns can have shivers sometimes. But if there is a tremor or shakiness regularly, see the baby's doctor.

Low blood sugar, low calcium level in the blood, and low vitamin D level can be the cause.

But it is important to know that there is no seizure activity.

Describe to the doctor exactly what happens.

Feeding

Breastfeeding. When it comes to feeding your baby, breastfeeding is preferred over formula. During the first few days after delivery, the small amount of breast milk produced is called colostrum. Colostrum is rich in immunoglobulins that help fight infections.

It takes three to four days or longer for the milk to come in, and during that time, the baby gets the colostrum. By that time, the baby will usually nurse for about ten minutes on each side. Initially the baby eats every two hours, then every three to four hours. Frequent feeding helps increase your milk supply.

While breastfeeding, it's important to keep the breast away from the baby's nostrils because babies breathe only through their nose. Be sure to clean the baby's nostrils if he or she has been congested by using a bulb syringe. Babies open their eyes when they begin to eat, and it's good to look into your baby's eyes and talk to him or her while breastfeeding.

Breastfeeding requires patience, particularly in the beginning when both mother and child are learning the process. Mothers are often tired and frustrated during the first few weeks. Babies usually cry at night, so mothers should do their best to sleep during the day. Once the adjustment period is over, breastfeeding is a rewarding and inexpensive way to feed a baby.

Keep a limit on the nursing time to thirty to forty minutes. If the mother becomes ill and has a high fever while nursing, she should stop breastfeeding temporarily. A mother can take Tylenol if needed to combat the fever. When resuming breastfeeding, wear a mask.

Here are a few guidelines to help mothers who are breastfeeding:

- Hand washing is an easy way to prevent illness.
- Avoid tobacco and alcohol.
- Eliminate gassy foods like cabbage, beans, and broccoli.
- Limit coffee, chocolate, and spicy foods.
- Stay hydrated.
- Eat foods that are high in vitamins and iron.

- Find a comfortable position for nursing by sitting with a straight back and leaning against a firm surface. Use a stool to prop up your feet.

Babies sometimes need extra fluids. You can give your baby Pedialyte or water. Tap water should be boiled first. You want to add a little sugar as well, one teaspoon per four ounces of water. Don't give your baby more than a couple of ounces of water a day.

If he or she needs more fluids, give Pedialyte.

Breast milk is low in vitamin D and iron; therefore, breastfed babies need to take vitamins with iron. Ask your baby's doctor about it. Even if you take vitamins, that will not provide enough vitamins for your baby.

Breasts can become sore as a result of breastfeeding. Here are a few ways to avoid soreness:

- Gradually increase the feeding time.
- Don't let the baby suck only on the nipple. Instead encourage the baby to suck on a larger part of the breast.
- If you have a sore, ask the obstetrician for a cream to improve healing. Be sure to remove the cream before nursing.
- Relieve engorged breasts by nursing and pumping.
- If the nipples are flat, try rubbing them before feeding.
- If the nipple is inverted or large, use a nipple shield or pump.
- If your breast is not only hard but also red and tender, see your obstetrician.

Breastfeeding is recommended until one year of age, but it can go longer.

Once a good nursing pattern has been established, you can wean gradually as many feedings as necessary while working. Give your baby pumped breast milk. That way you can continue to keep your baby on breast milk. Breast milk can be stored in the freezer for months or in the refrigerator for forty-eight hours. After your baby drinks from a bottle, it cannot be reused.

To prevent waste, try to put only as much milk in a bottle as the baby typically drinks during one feeding.

The breast pump should be completely dismantled and washed in the dishwasher. Containers used for breast milk go to the dishwasher as well. Do not use chemical disinfection. Do not use a microwave. Frozen milk that was thawed should not be used longer than two hours. Use glass containers, not plastic.

Situations in which it is harmful to breastfeed. There are situations where breastfeeding can be harmful because of certain diseases and medications. These situations are called contraindications.

Contraindications for breastfeeding:

- If the mother has tuberculosis.
- If the mother has HIV.
- If the mother has herpes infection and the blisters are located on the mother's breasts.
- If the mother is using drugs.
- If the baby has galactosemia (galactosemia is a genetic metabolic disorder that affects an individual's ability to metabolize the sugar galactose properly). This disorder is detected by the newborn screening test that is done in the newborn nursery and at the two weeks office visit.
- When the mother is sick with a very high fever. After the fever subsides, breastfeeding can be resumed. However, the mother needs to wear a face mask while nursing or holding the baby. Pump your breast while the high fever lasts.

If the mother has a breast infection, she still can nurse.

Many pharmaceutical drugs are safe for breastfeeding mothers to take, if necessary. But there are drugs harmful for babies. Mothers cannot take these drugs while breastfeeding. If they have to take any of those medications, breastfeeding needs to be stopped.

These harmful medications include the following:

- Laxatives
- Blood thinners or anticoagulants
- Cancer medications and antimetabolites
- Certain birth control pills. Consult your ob-gyn
- Headache medications that are ergot alkaloids like sumatriptan or Imitrex

- Medications for a hyperactive thyroid gland which are called antithyroid drugs
- Iodide which is used to treat certain thyroid diseases
- Certain mental health medications like lithium
- Drugs to treat parasites, like metronidazole
- Strong opioid painkillers like morphine, tramadol, oxycodone, fentanyl, methadone, meperidine, and Dilaudid
- Radiopharmaceuticals like radioactive iodine

Have a question about medication? You can ask your doctor or the baby's pediatrician about what pharmaceuticals are safe to take while breastfeeding.

Formula feeding

Formula feeding generally begins with a cow's-milk-based formula, but there are exceptions. Families with a history of a milk allergy or intolerance, or in cases in which the baby has difficulty processing the formula, a cow's-milk-based formula can be substituted with a soy or elemental formula. Premature babies are usually fed with a formula that has more calories.

Formulas come in a variety of forms: powder, liquid, concentrate, or ready to feed. As long as you prepare the formula exactly according to the directions, then it shouldn't matter which form you use. Only use boiled water when preparing the formula. Formulas already contain vitamins including vitamin D. It also has iron, so usually no extra vitamins or iron are needed. Even so, breast feeding is still superior and desirable.

It's a good idea to stick with the formula your baby tolerates. After a baby drinks from a bottle, don't reuse that bottle until it's been washed with boiling water (sterilized).

Newborns may not be too eager to eat on the first and second day after delivery. Generally, during the first week, they eat one to two ounces every three hours. Gradually, babies will eat more, and feedings will be once every three to four hours. Newborns with low birth weights will need more frequent feedings, like every two hours.

Give your baby as much formula as he or she wants, not as much as you think is needed. Do not push the baby to eat or to finish a bottle. If the baby is healthy, he or she will eat enough. You shouldn't give your baby more than thirty-two ounces of formula per day. Some parents believe that heavy babies are healthier, but pediatricians actually prefer babies to be proportional.

Formula feeding no-nos:

- Don't let your baby sleep with the bottle—this can cause choking and damage to the baby's teeth.
- Don't prop the bottle up.
- Avoid whole milk until the baby is a year old.

Preparing for your newborn's first office visit

The best time for the first appointment is one to two days after your baby was discharged from the nursery.

This way the doctor can follow up on problems like jaundice.

Take the baby's discharge papers from the hospital with you.

The doctor will check the baby thoroughly to be sure everything is okay.

Try to make the appointment at a time when the office is not busy or when it is a set time for healthy babies. It is good to take another person with you, like the father, a relative, or a trusted friend who knows how to take care of a baby.

Write down your questions and concerns before the visit. Take your insurance card with you and any documents you got from the hospital.

When you are in the waiting room, try to stay away from others.

Take with you extra cloth, diapers, wipes, diaper cream, and pacifier. Do not have the pacifier on a string around the baby's neck. If your baby is on formula, take a bottle with you. Also take a blanket, and keep the baby warm all the time.

Before you see the doctor, the baby's weight, height, and head circumference will be measured. These measurements will be done at every healthy visit and marked on the growth chart (see growth chart).

This is the way the doctor can follow the baby's growth.

Newborns usually lose weight after birth. After that, there is a rapid weight gain, and he or she gains two pounds by one month of age, then about one pound a month.

The doctor also regularly follows the baby's development (see development).

Another appointment is necessary at two weeks of age, when the second newborn screening test is done. The first one was done in the nursery.

Well-baby and well-child routine visit schedule, showing the ages when a doctor visit is important

These are the ages when a doctor visit is necessary.

- 2 days
- 2 weeks
- 1 month
- 2 month
- 4 month
- 6 month
- 9 month
- 12 month
- 15 month
- 18 month
- 2 years
- 3 years
- 4 years

After 4 years, there are annual visits.

The visits usually include the following:

- measurements of height, weight, and head circumference (for the baby) as well
- history and physical exam
- following of development
- discussion of feeding and diet
- keeping immunizations up to date
- anticipatory guidance (preparing the parents for antici-pated development; it also includes age-specific teaching about injury and disease prevention)
- answering of your questions and concerns
- screening tests for certain diseases

- (for adolescents) discussion of the physical and sexual changes and healthy lifestyle (including alcohol, tobacco smoking, and sex)

It will be helpful for you write down all your questions and concerns ahead.

C. *Beyond the newborn period*

Solid foods. Solid foods like cereals, vegetables, and fruits are usually introduced to a formula-fed baby when he or she is between four and six months old. Breastfed babies will generally begin eating solid foods at six months of age. Discuss the specifics of feeding with the doctor.

The first solid food is typically cereal, such as oatmeal, rice, barley. If the baby is always hungry and wants to eat more than thirty-two ounces of formula per day, then you might introduce cereal before the baby is four months old. Keep in mind that rice cereal will make a baby's stools harder, while barley cereal will make them softer.

After cereal, the next step is vegetables. It's a good idea to introduce veggies before fruits. If fruits are introduced first, then the baby might refuse vegetables because they aren't as sweet. In terms of jarred food, strained vegetables are a good start. Yellow vegetables are often the starting point. Many babies enjoy sweet potatoes as a first vegetable.

Foods should gradually be incorporated into your baby's diet one step at the time. When you start to introduce vegetables, use first-stage food, then the second stage once the baby is six months old, and the third stage at about nine months old. Start with small portions, and slowly increase to a full feeding. The amount of milk he or she drinks decreases as the solids increase. Stick with the same vegetable for a few days before beginning a new one. The golden rule: increase the amounts gradually, and only make one change at a time.

If you're making your own baby food, it should be very thin first, then gradually increase the food's coarseness as the baby gets older. Don't add sugar or salt to your baby's food.

Carrots contain nitrates, and that can cause a disorder called *methemoglobinemia* (see methemoglobinemia). Therefore, do not make your own carrot. Feed your baby with carrot baby food that you buy instead. At six months, two different vegetables are recommended, and you can introduce meat. When preparing your own baby food, mix only a small amount of well-grounded meat into a vegetable. The best meat to start with is chicken. Double-check your baby's food, and make sure there aren't any bones or chunky pieces.

Avoid desserts, and be cautious around eggs. Don't introduce eggs until your baby is a year old. Scrambled eggs, for example, can cause a severe allergic reaction.

When your baby is ten months old, he or she can start to nibble on table foods like mashed potatoes and mushy vegetables. After a year, your baby can start eating table food. A parent should always be with a baby when he or she is eating, to prevent choking. Foods that can cause choking include pieces of apples, grapes, carrots, celery, seeds, meat, and hot dogs. Do not give nuts, popcorn, hard candies, gum in the first three years.

Introduce juice after twelve months of age. Serve only 100 percent fruit juice, not juice drinks. Limit the juice to two fluid ounces per day.

Do not give honey until the baby passes the first birthday because it can cause a severe disease called *botulism*.

Botulism is caused by bacteria called *clostridium botulinum*. This germ can be present in honey, (also in Karo syrup) and produces a toxin affecting the nervous system.

Symptoms are generalized weakness and paralysis that can lead to respiratory failure.

Therapy: supportive care, *clostridium botulism* immune globulin

In the first year:

- No egg white, because it can cause an allergic reaction.
- No honey, because it can cause a serious disease botulism (see above).
- No juice, because fruit juice offers no nutritional benefit at this age but extra sugar, and that can cause tooth decay. Do not give juices to your child at bedtime. Generally, whole fruit juices are recommended. Limit the amount of juice for toddlers to two to four ounces daily, children four to six ounces per day.

- No whole milk, because of the risk of allergy and anemia (see anemia).

Discuss the baby's feeding with the doctor.

Preparing for a visit to the pediatrician.

It is good to write down your questions and concerns ahead of time.

With every symptom in my book, I wrote down questions your pediatrician probably will ask. You can prepare the answers to those questions before the visit.

Take the medications that your child takes with you.

It helps to take your child's favorite book and toy with you for possible waiting and if you need to calm him down.

Talk to your child before the visit so he knows what to expect, and prepare him for shots (see attitudes).

Owning a doctor's kit can make your child more familiar with the visit.

Growth and development/growth charts.

It is important for your baby and child to have regular checkups. During healthy checkups, the baby's height, weight, and head circumference are measured, and the development is checked.

For children, the height, weight, and development are looked at.

Growth charts are used to evaluate the height and weight of babies and children. Also the head circumference of babies is measured by placing a tape measure around their head.

These charts are useful tools to compare the measurements of individual infants and children of the same age. They track the height and weight of children from zero to eighteen years of age. There is a different chart for girls and boys. The comparison is given by percentage. The curves of the growth chart show whether the height and weight of an individual baby or child and the head circumference of a baby are in the normal range. Another important role of the growth chart is to show whether a baby or child grows and gains weight properly and the head circumference increases the way it is supposed to.

It also shows how the height and weight relate to each other, how proportional the child is. The height and weight do not have to be in the same percentage, but they have to be in the normal range. The closer the percentage of the height and weight are, the more proportional the child is.

There is a growth chart for premature babies as well, from twenty-two to fifty weeks, in weekly increments.

Babies usually grow one-half to one inch per month and gain about one pound per month in the first year. They gain more in the first month. The height increase is about half of the height at birth by twelve months of age. The weight usually doubles at six months and triples at twelve months. The height and weight of premature babies lags behind, and they usually catch up by two years of age.

Babies who were small for gestational age (SGA) are also shorter than other term babies.

During the second year, a toddler grows about four to five inches per year, while between two to six years, the growth is three inches per year.

From six to twelve years, the average growth is about two and a half inches.

During puberty, there is a rapid growth (growth spurt).

The weight gain between two and three years of age is five to six pounds. Between three and five years, the yearly weight gain is four to six pounds.

From six to twelve years, the weight gain is about seven pounds per year. During puberty, there is a faster weight gain.

One of the most common questions for pediatricians is, When will my baby do this or that? Many parents have questions about their baby's development like: When will my baby roll over? Sit up? Crawl? Stand up? Talk? When will his or her teeth come in? Is my baby's development normal?

There are no easy answers to these questions because the age when a baby or toddler will reach a new *developmental milestone* can vary. Here are a few average markers:

Two months old

- Babies can usually follow lights and respond to noises.
- Babies start to smile spontaneously.

Four months old

- Babies learn to roll over.
- Babies can find objects accidentally but might not grab them.
- Babies start to laugh and squeal.

Six months old

- Babies sit up.

- Babies can reach and grab objects.
- Teething often begins, usually with lower scissors.

Nine months old

- Babies begin to stand up (this can happen before sitting up).
- Babies will start making sounds that resemble words like "da-da-da" or "ma-ma-ma."

One year old

- They can stand on their own and begin walking, taking one or two steps.
- They start speaking more clearly and saying "mama," "dada," and maybe another word.
- Molars may start to form, although the process might take longer.

Fifteen months old

- They can walk well, drink from cup, imitate housework, and can say two to three words besides "mama" and "dada."

Two years old

- They can use spoon spilling a little, dump raisin from a bottle, scribble, point to a couple of named body parts, kick the ball forward, combine two words.

Three years old

- They can copy a circle, build a tower with four cubes, follow directions, name pictures, put on some clothing, wash and dry hands, kick the ball, throw it overhand, balance on

one foot for one second, broad jump, walk up stairs with alternating legs, pedal tricycle, speak short sentences, use plurals.
- Many three-year-olds are toilet-trained.

Four years old

- They can copy a cross, maybe a square, build a tower of eight cubes, comprehend cold, hungry, tired, recognize colors, button up, dress with little help, understand prepositions such as above, under, on, etc.

Five years old

- They can separate from their mother easily, draw recognizable man, balance on one foot for five seconds, hop on one foot, catch bounced balls, heel to toe walk, know opposite analogies like ice is cold, fire is hot, elephant is big, mouth is small, give first and last name.

Other common questions include: What will my baby's eye color look like? Be patient. Eye color can change for many months.

Parents are naturally anxious if they believe that their child's development is slower compared to their peers. Don't panic, development greatly varies between different children.

Your pediatrician will check your child's development.

Talk to your baby frequently, look in her eyes, and smile at her. Touch her, read to her, sing to her if you can, and have her listen to music. All of these things can help her development.

D. Children

Toddlers (one to two years). During the second year, toddlers are moving around more and aware of themselves and their surroundings. They want to explore more things. They want more independence, and "no" becomes a favorite word. They imitate others and start to put two words together.

After one year of age, the child's food intake often decreases. A baby usually triples his weight in the first year and gains less in subsequent years. If the weight is okay, there is no reason to worry.

Two to three years. After two years, the appetite increases. Sometimes a child refuses a meal, particularly if it is a new one. By this time, he eats table food. Actually, after one year, the child mostly eats what others eat in the family. But you need to be careful to cut up the food to small pieces and be sure that he does not eat chunky food, does not bite off a piece of apple, carrots, celery, or hot dogs. Also that he does not get nuts, fruits with seeds, like cherry and whole grape, popcorn, candy, or gum because they are choking hazards. It is important to eat a healthy, well-balanced diet with plenty of fruits and vegetables.

At two years of age, it is time for toilet training, if the child is ready (see toilet training).

Speech and movements are gradually improving.

By the age of two to three, he likes to help undressing and dressing and brushing his teeth.

Start toothbrushing early, as soon as your child has the first teeth. Use very tiny toothpaste so he does not swallow it.

He likes to build with blocks and manipulate objects.

At age three, he probably can ride a tricycle.

Preschoolers (three to five years). They try to discover more and more about their surroundings, and that often puts them in danger. It is important to childproof the home at this time, if it has not been done before (see safety advises).

They have better coordination and like running, climbing, and jumping. They love to go to the playground. Be careful, and always watch your child closely.

Three to five years. They are interested in other children and to play with them. They can start nursery school. Speech improves a great deal, and they can express themselves better and better. They like to play games, and they like to play with balls. Their movement is more coordinated. They like to color and learn to use scissors. They start preschool, then kindergarten, and that is a big change for them.

Five to six years. Children start school at this age, but play is still important. They play with other children and learn to share things. Their attention span is longer. They talk more, and the sentences get more complicated. Their coordination improves, and they can learn how to ride a bike and catch a ball. Their motor skill improves, and they learn how to tie shoelaces, use zips, and button up.

School-age children (six to twelve years)

Six to seven years. They enjoy more activities and probably can ride a bike. They cooperate and share more. They like board games. They start to make friends.

Seven to eight years. They have friends and learn new things in school.

Eight to nine years. They completely dress themselves.

Nine to twelve years. They read well, maybe write stories. They draw, paint, and can use tools. They have multiple friends, often a best friend.

They play more sports, often team sports, maybe organized sports. Sport injuries are more common when playing team sports. Children have growth plates in the bones, and they are vulnerable to stress. Growth plates are areas of growing tissues close to the end of the long bones in the arms and legs of children and adolescents.

Symptoms of growth plate injury are pain, inability to put weight or pressure on the limb, or move it.

If your child has these symptoms, do not let him bear weight on the limb, and go to the emergency room.

Treatment is splint or cast. If the bone is out of place, it needs to be put back (it is called reduction). In case of severe injury, surgery may be necessary.

Sprains, strains, and fractures are the most common injuries. Overuse injuries are not uncommon, when repetitive movements put stress on the same body part. *Stress fractures* and ligament tears can occur (see fractures).

Anterior cruciate ligament (ACL) injury is most common in sports that involve sudden stops and turns. The ACL is the ligament connecting the thigh bone (femur) to the shinbone (tibia).

Prevention of sport injuries:

- The child needs to understand the rules of the sport.
- Use appropriate equipment.
- If the child is overly tired or has pain, he needs to take a break.
- If the child suffers an injury, he should not continue to play or reenter the game.
- The child should be in good shape before he starts an organized sport.

It is important that child and adolescent athletes eat a high carbohydrate meal three to four hours before training or a game. Also, they need a high-calorie snack one to two hours before the training.

They need to drink plenty of fluids before, during, and after the activity. They need more fluids in hot weather because they sweat more.

After the training or game, they need more carbohydrates and proteins. Naturally, fat, vitamins, and iron also need to be included in the diet.

It is important to find a balance between academics and sports.

E. Adolescents (see puberty)

This is a time of great physical growth, sexual development, and the development of abstract thinking.

Adolescents need more calories and larger food portions. Discourage junk foods.

It is important to avoid sport injuries and prevent heat exhaustion and heat stroke (see heat and cold related illnesses). For nutrition with sport events, see above.

Girls start their menstrual period (see menstrual period, menstrual problems).

Accurate sex education is important since many adolescents are sexually active. They need to know about birth control and the prevention of sexually transmitted diseases (STD) (see sexually transmitted diseases and sex education).

Transfer to adult care. When you or your child thinks that he or she needs to change from the pediatrician to a new doctor who treats adults, whether your child is eighteen or twenty-one years old, you want to select one. When you have found a doctor, have your child's medical records transferred. Be sure to have a current immunization record.

Prepare for the first visit with the doctor. He needs to know your child's medical history, all the diseases he had, particularly if there is any ongoing problem. He or she needs to know all the allergies your child has, and most importantly, drug allergies. If he takes medications, take them with you.

The family history is also important.

Advice, concern, safety

You spend most of your time taking care of the new baby. You feed him or her, comfort your baby, change the diapers several times a day. It is no wonder your other child or children, particularly the younger ones, can get jealous. They feel that you only care about the new baby. So try to spend as much time as possible with your other child or children. If dad spends more time with them, that helps but does not substitute for the mom. It is also a good idea that when you go home from the hospital, have a present for the young sister or brother, and tell them that the new baby brought it. If your other child or children are jealous, watch them closely to be sure they do not harm the baby.

Prepare your child or children ahead of time for the birth of the new baby. Tell your child about the time when he or she was a baby. Show your child photos. Involve your child in preparations for the new baby.

Keep your dog and cat away from the new baby because they can hurt him or her.

Keep your infant on his back when sleeping, not on the stomach or on the side. But if you closely watch your baby, he or she can have some tummy time.

When you pick up your baby, always hold the head and the neck. When you bathe him, hold his arm so he does not slip.

When you change your baby's diaper, be sure that you have everything at hand you need so you do not need to make even a step. Do not leave your baby unattended for a second when you fetch for things.

Keep your baby in your room for at least the first six months of life, preferably for the first year. Again, he or she should sleep on the back in the crib. The mattress should be firm. Keep soft objects, pillows, stuffed animals out of the crib to prevent suffocation and *sudden infant death syndrome (SIDS)*, now called *sudden unexpected infant death (SUID)*. The use of inclined sleepers, in bed sleepers, soft padding, crib bumpers, loungers, travel sleepers, and compact sleepers, are not recommended because of the same safety reasons.

If you use a sling, be sure it fits well and the baby is safe. Check your baby often to see that the neck is straight and the sling does not block the baby's nose and mouth. Be sure that the baby cannot fall out of the sling even when you bend down and that he cannot slip through the holes.

Do not use sling if your baby is premature or had respiratory problems. Do not sleep in the same bed with your baby, because you can injure him or her. Products that are for bed sharing are not safe either. Never leave your baby on your bed. Even if you put pillows around him, he still can fall off.

Be sure that nobody shakes your baby because strong shaking can cause brain damage. Keep your baby warm in cold weather. Avoid exposure of your child's face to cold weather and direct contact to cold objects. Exposure to cold can cause local injury and rash. Be careful if the weather is hot because he or she can have heat-related injuries (see heat- and cold-related injuries).

Do not leave strollers and car seats in the sun because such exposures can cause burns.

For babies, it is best to avoid direct sun exposure. Keep your baby in the shade. If there is no shade, you can use an umbrella. But watch your baby, because he can get sunburn when the position of the sun changes. Dress him in protective clothing—a hat with a brim and sunglasses. If your baby is older than six months, you can use sunscreen. Use sunscreen that contains zinc oxide, and reapply it every two hours or more often if your baby is in the water. Use sunscreen that does not contain benzene, oxybenzone, and avobenzone.

When you bathe your baby, check the bathwater temperature with your elbow to be sure it is not too hot. Always hold his arm firmly so he will not slide. Do not use a bath seat because that can be dangerous. The infant can fall out of the seat. For water safety, do not leave your baby or young child in the bathtub alone, not even for a second. Have everything that you need for the bathing, including a towel and the baby's cloth, within arm's length.

The milk that you give your baby can be room temperature, but if you warm it, be sure it has the right temperature.

Be sure you never leave your baby or child alone in the car, not even for a minute.

You want to make your house babyproof and childproof. Cover the sharp edges of the furniture, and remove items from areas the baby might reach.

Always have the side rails of the bed up. Install a safety rail at the stairs, and keep the gate closed to prevent your baby or toddler going to the stairs. Be sure that the gate is safe, that the baby's or toddler's neck cannot be entrapped and he or she cannot fit under the gate to pass it.

Do not leave your infant or toddler alone. Beware that your baby can easily fall out of a high chair.

It is okay to use pacifiers. But do not fasten the pacifier with a string to his cloth or put it around his neck, because that can cause choking. Do not put necklaces on the baby or toddler for the same reason.

Do not put a ring on the baby's hand, because injury can occur if the ring remains stuck on the hold when the baby falls.

Do not smoke or have anything hot in your hand when holding the baby, because you can cause burns.

Always feed your baby or toddler in a sitting position, and stay there while he or she is eating.

In the first year, do not give the baby the following:

- egg white
- honey
- juice
- whole milk
- Karo syrup

Do not give honey or Karo syrup to your baby during the first year because it can cause a severe, life-threatening disease called botulism. The cause is a bacteria clostridium botulinum that produces a toxin that absorbs from the baby's bowels.

Symptoms are constipation, weak cry, difficulty sucking, poor muscle tone (the baby is floppy), and paralysis.

If the baby has these symptoms, go to the emergency room or call 911.

Do not give your baby or toddler nuts, popcorn, candy, gum, grapes, or a piece of apple, carrot, celery, or hot dog, because of choking hazard. Do not let him walk or run while eating. Keep him away from coins, thumbtacks, paperclips, and any small objects for the same reason. Small batteries are particularly dangerous. If a battery is swallowed, go to the emergency room right away.

Give your child a healthy, well-balanced diet.

That includes proteins like meat, dairy products, eggs, and mushrooms. Beans, lentil, soy, and peanut butter are also high in protein. Yogurt is very healthy.

Carbohydrates like cereal, bread, pasta, potatoes, rice.

Vegetables, fruits. Include as much in the diet as possible. Wash them thoroughly with a strong stream of running water several times. Also rub them.

Do not give your child too much fried food, red meat, or eggs. Keep junk food to an absolute minimum.

Eating too much sugar or salt is not healthy.

Have your child drink plenty of fluids, but offer drinks containing sugar, like sodas, only rarely, and even juice should be given only once a day. There is nothing wrong with drinking water.

For everyone who keeps a vegetarian or vegan diet, multivitamins are recommended. Talk to the doctor.

Try to have family dinners every night. That is the time when you can talk to your child or children without TV or cell phones or other distractions.

Be sure your child has a good night's sleep. It is important to develop a good night time routine (see the chapter on sleep: sleep problems).

Limit the time your child spends in front of the TV, playing video games, or using the cell phone. The total time should not be more than two hours a day. Less is better. No screen under two years of age. It is okay to say no to your child. That is part of child-rearing.

It is also good to see that he or she watches age-appropriate material.

Have your child exercise regularly for at least one hour daily and spend some time outside. Also, children need to have time to play. Use plenty of sunscreen. SPF should be at least thirty, but fifty or above fifty is preferable.

The first appointment with an eye doctor is recommended at one year of age. Your child needs another appointment at age three and five. After five years of age, visit the eye doctor every one to two years, but preferably every year.

Teach your child personal hygiene, like washing up, brushing teeth, and flossing. Flossing is very important. Visit the dentist every six months.

Be sure your child washes his or her hands every time after using the toilet, before meals, and after coming home.

Teach your child a good toilet routine. It is important to urinate at least four times a day and have a bowel movement daily. Have your child sit on the toilet every day at the same time.

You can start toilet training around two years of age. But if your child is not ready, wait longer. Be patient.

Teach your daughter that after using the toilet, she has to wipe herself from front to back and not go back with the same toilet paper to prevent urinary tract infection.

Develop a daily routine that your child will follow.

For the protection of your child's eyes, do not let him read in dim light. Have your child get at least two hours of sunlight daily (even sitting by a window is good). These measures seem to have a protective effect against nearsightedness.

Excessive screen time can affect your child's eyes. Teach your child the 20-20-20 rule. Every twenty minutes, look away from the screen for twenty seconds, and focus on something at least twenty feet away.

It is useful to take a break every hour.

Teenagers should use contact lenses properly. Be sure she does not wear them when sleeping or swimming. The solution she keeps the lens in should not be reused. The lenses should not be cleaned with tap water.

Teach your child not to listen to the radio, TV, computer, mobile phone, or CDs too loud. Teenagers like to listen to loud music, and that can harm their hearing. If your child plays an instrument, particularly the drums, have him wear a proper earplug.

Your child should not play with turtles because he can contract salmonella infection, causing diarrhea (see diarrhea).

Teach your child to be aware of animals and strangers.

Keep distance from unfamiliar animals.

Teach him to back away slowly from animals.

Prevent your child from provoking or playing rough with a dog.

Your child should not stay behind a horse, because the horses kick backward.

Teach your child not to eat plants, colorful berries, or mushrooms that you did not give him or her.

Have the telephone number of Poison Control easily accessible.

Poison Control Centers telephone number: 1-800-222-1222.

Teach your child early on not to cross the road without you. He needs to learn how to look around when crossing the road and learn how the traffic lights work.

Do not let your child ride off-road vehicles before sixteen years of age. Be sure he wears helmet, and never drives on paved road. There should be no driving without a driver's license. He needs to be careful with golf carts.

If your child rides a bicycle or uses a scooter, skateboard, Segway, roller skates, Rollerblades, ice skates, skis, snowboard, or horse rides, be sure he or she wears an appropriate helmet that follows US government standards. Parents should always wear helmets when biking as well to set a good example for their children. Infants in bicycle baskets also should wear helmets. Also use protective pads, goggles, and mouth guards to prevent injuries.

Hoverboards are dangerous.

Do not let your child use a trampoline without a trainer because injuries are common.

Teach your child your address and telephone number as soon as possible. Also teach him whom to turn to if he gets lost.

Teach him the proper use of 911.

Be sure to buy toys that do not have loose pieces that a young child can remove. Again, think about the battery in the toys. Children also put small objects, like beans, green peas, corn, etc., in their nose and ears, and girls to their vagina. Try to prevent that.

Be sure your child does not eat dirt and paint chips because that can cause lead poisoning (see poisonings). But if you see your child eating those things or any nonfood items, see the doctor.

Eating nonfood items might be associated with anemia.

Plastic bags can be dangerous too. The child can put the bag over his head, and the bag can cause suffocation. Also, he or she can swallow a piece of the plastic bag and choke. A piece of rubber gloves and balloons can also cause choking. If you have a rubber glove from the doctor's office, be sure to throw it away before you leave.

Always keep electric cords in good shape. Have a smoke alarm, carbon monoxide detector, and a fire extinguisher.

Young children most often suffer electric injuries when they bite into electric cords or poke metals into the outlets.

The burn can be localized only at the mouth or can be more serious.

Children should be protected around sports equipment, because they can cause severe injuries. Young children need to be supervised at all times around sports equipment. Exercise machines should not be in areas where children play. They should be unplugged when not used. Exercise rooms should be locked.

Lightning and high voltage can cause severe organ injuries and can stop the heart beating. Severe neurologic injury can occur as well.

If the child comes in contact with electricity, pull the plug right away. If that is not possible, remove the wire with a dry thick nonmetal object. Do not touch the child, because you can get electrocuted.

If the heart stops, start cardiopulmonary resuscitation (CPR) immediately, and call 911.

Keep electric outlets covered, and keep your child away from electrical cords to prevent burns. Teach your child that during storms, it is best to stay inside. Be sure that your child comes out of the pool or any natural water at once and does not touch any metal object. He needs to know not to stay under a tree during a storm. Watch your young child closely in the kitchen so he or she does not get close to a hot oven, a hot pot, or hot liquids. Also prevent him or her from touching hot iron or curling iron.

Be sure that your young child does not play on the balcony, does not have access to an open window, and cannot open the window. Also watch that your child does not climb too high on the monkey bars or on a tree and does not jump from a moving swing.

Prevent your child from going to the pool alone. The best prevention is a fence around the pool that can be locked. Have a fence that surrounds four sides of the pool and has a gate that is self-closing and self-latching.

Have your child learn to swim early on. All infants, toddlers, young children and anybody who is not a good swimmer should wear life jackets when near water.

Adults should supervise children in pools and natural waters within arm's length and without any distractions (food, drink, reading, games, telephones, etc.). Do not leave your child under the supervision of another child.

Children and adolescents need to wear approved life jackets when boating.

Also be careful with any large containers that hold any liquids, because of the drowning hazard.

Keep your small child away from tools and sharp objects, including knives and forks.

Do not let your young child stay in the garage alone, and be sure that he or she does not have access to the garage door opener. Keep the car keys in a safe place.

Do not let your child play in and around vehicles. Always keep the car doors and the trunk locked.

Always use a car seat and booster seat until your child grows out of it. Use an approved car seat, and be sure that it is correctly anchored. Infants and toddlers should be in the back seat in a car and facing backward as long as possible. That is the safest way to travel in the car. When your infant outgrows the rear-facing-only car seat, he needs a convertible seat that is rear-facing (around two years). Children under thirteen years of age should be in the rear seat. In the front seat, children can sustain very severe injuries from inflating air bag. Do not install rear-facing car seat there either because of the same reason. It is not safe to have your child sit on your lap. Your child needs to learn that the first thing when sitting in the car is to buckle up.

As I mentioned before, never leave your child in the car alone, not for a minute.

If your child goes to the woods, have him wear long-sleeved shirts, long pants, a hat, and closed shoes to avoid tick bites. To avoid mosquito bites, use repellents, and do not stay outside at dawn and dusk. If using repellents, be sure that it does not get in the eyes or mouth. Do not let your water hose drip because that draws mosquitoes.

Teach your child to be careful with a campfire. Do not let your child play with fireworks because injuries are common, particularly eye injuries and injury to the thumb. The loss of the thumb can occur.

Keep matches in a safe place.

Use regular and not antiseptic soap, unless a doctor recommends it. Regular use of antiseptic soaps can make the germs stronger. When your child takes a bath, do not use a bubble bath because it can cause irritation. Girls should not use tight underpants.

If any chemical gets into the child's eyes, wash it with water for a few minutes, then go to the emergency room.

For food safety, avoid processed meats, particularly during pregnancy. Eating fresh or frozen fruits and vegetables is very important. Do not warm foods and beverages in plastic containers because potentially harmful substances, like bisphenol A (BPA) and phthalates can get into the food. That includes pumped breast milk and formula. Do not put plastics in the dishwasher. Prefer the use of glass and stainless steel instead of plastic. Look at the recycling code on the bottom of products to see the type of the plastic. Avoid plastics with recycling codes 3 (phthalates), 6 (sterene), and 7 (bisphenols). Encourage good handwashing before handling foods and drinks.

Naturally, it is important to give your child the right medicine and the right dose. So always read the label before you give medication. If the medicine is a liquid, give it with a syringe or measuring spoon, not with a measuring cup.

Definitely do not put medicine or even vitamins in a bottle of milk or other liquid because there is no way to know how much medicine or vitamin the child gets.

Do not put medicine in an unlabeled container.

Do not mix medications together.

If the direction is every eight hours, that means three times a day. Every six hours means four times a day.

When your child goes to see the doctor, it is good practice to take all the medicines he or she takes with you.

While some medications come in liquid form, others come in drops. The drops are more concentrated.

So if accidentally drops are given in an amount as if it was a liquid, a medicine overdose can occur. Do not give any medicine more often than recommended. Even if your child has a fever and you have already given the Tylenol or ibuprofen or both and the temperature is still high, you cannot repeat that dose.

But in this case, you can give your child a sponge bath with lukewarm water to get the fever down.

Acetaminophen (Tylenol) cannot be given more often than every four hours and maximum five times over twenty-four hours. Ibuprofen (Motrin, Advil) cannot be given more often than every six hours, maximum four times a day. Give these medications only when you need them for fever or pain, and try not to give them for a long period of time because that can be harmful. Chronic use of acetaminophen can affect the liver, and chronic use of ibuprofen can hurt the kidneys. Do not give them to the child for a simple cold without fever. If the temperature is 102.5 Fahrenheit or above, give ibuprofen. Otherwise give Tylenol if the temperature is 100 degrees Fahrenheit or above. But if the child gets seizures with fever, give Tylenol or Motrin above 99.6 degrees Fahrenheit.

If you need to use either of these medications longer than two days, call the doctor.

If you need to give "cold" medicine to your child, check the label to be sure you know if it has acetaminophen or ibuprofen. That way if the child has fever, you do not give a double dose of these medicines. Do not give cold medicine to a child under six years of age.

Do not give aspirin to your child unless it was ordered by a doctor. It can cause a severe disease called *Reye's syndrome* (see common cold "Flu").

If the child vomits the medicine you gave, do not repeat it, but wait for the next dose when it is due.

If he or she vomits the medicine a second time, call the doctor.

If your child takes antibiotics, give him or her a probiotic ordered by the doctor or plain yogurt daily to prevent possible side effects like diarrhea caused by a germ *clostridium difficile or C. diff.* The yogurt should contain "good bacteria" like lactobacillus. You can flavor it.

Do not use pain reducer like local tooth liquid, spray, or gel products under age two, because it contains benzocaine and can cause a severe disease called *methemoglobinemia* (see methemoglobinemia).

Do not give more vitamins to your child than recommended. Vitamin overdose can be harmful (see vitamins).

In case of accidental ingestion of a medicine, call your child's doctor, Poison Control Center, or go to the emergency room. Again, have the telephone number of the Poison Control displayed in a place where you can find it at once.

If there is an accidental ingestion of chemicals, go to the emergency room, or call 911 right away.

If there is choking, a problem with breathing, color change (bluish color of the lips, around the lips, face, nail beds, or an extremely white color), seizure, or change of consciousness, call 911.

Medications and chemicals need to be locked and stored in a place the child cannot reach. Teach your child early on to take medications only when necessary. Children should not drink coffee, regular tea, or alcohol and should not take stimulants, energy drinks, diet pills, and performance-enhancing substances like steroids. You want your child to know about the dangers of drugs, alcohol, and tobacco in any form. Try not to let your child associate with children who use these substances.

Electronic cigarettes are as dangerous as regular cigarettes.

Keep electronic cigarette packages that look like food away from children. Vaping and juuling is also tobacco smoking.

It is very important for your child to learn the dangers of drinking and driving. He needs to know not to sit in a car if the driver is not sober or taking any drug. The same is true of a driver texting or using a cellphone.

Your teenager needs to know the value of using a condom to prevent sexually transmitted diseases and pregnancies.

Your child needs to be aware of bees, wasps, hornets, etc.

If your child has an allergy, be sure that he or she has EpiPen (epinephrine) at home, in school, and camp.

Gun safety. Firearms are a significant cause of injury and death among children and adolescents.

If there is a gun in the home, preventative measures are extremely important:

- Keep the gun unloaded.
- Keep the gun securely locked.
- Store the guns and ammunition in separate places and both locked.
- Never let your child know where the keys are, and keep them in a safe place.

- When handling the gun, never leave it unattended, not for a second.
- Use trigger lock.
- If your child goes to a friend, be sure his parents follow the same precautions, because injuries often occur in a friend's house.

The above precautions should be kept as well if you have a teenager at home, particularly since teens have a higher rate of suicide.

Attitude

It is important how you prepare your child for a visit to the pediatrician, and particularly for the most feared event—getting a shot.

Different parents handle the situation differently.

I heard some mothers tell their child, "The mean doctor will give you a shot." It was said somewhat jokingly, but the frightened child hears only that the doctor is mean and will hurt him. So the child will always be worried when going to a doctor. If the child feels animosity toward doctors, it will be carried over to adulthood. So he or she may not seek medical care even when it is necessary.

I also heard some mothers telling their child when he or she starts whining, "You will not get a shot." The next minute, the child gets a shot.

I also heard a parent saying, "I will not let the doctor hurt you." The child gets the shot right after that. In these cases, the child will not trust the mother in the future.

It is very different when mothers tell their child, "The shot will hurt a little, but you will be all right. The doctor is your friend. You need to get the shot to keep you healthy. It will protect you against very bad diseases." If the child knows that the doctor wants to do what is best, he or she will trust doctors in the future. The child will know that if something is done that hurts, it is done for his or her best interest.

By the way, it helps if you draw your child's attention by talking to him or her or asking him or her to blow in the air like blowing out a candle while getting the shot.

It is also good to take with you your child's favorite toy, or "trusted friend," like a toy bear. Getting a doctor's kit also can help. Your child can examine you, a sibling, or a doll, bear, etc. Also, he or she can give shots.

Circumcision

Circumcision is the surgical removal of the skin covering the tip of the penis.

It is a rather common procedure for newborn boys in the US. Circumcision is done for religious, cultural, health reasons, or because it is a family tradition.

Circumcision is usually done in the newborn nursery.

Local anesthetic is used before the procedure.

The benefits of circumcision are the following:

- Easy cleaning of the penis
- No problem with phimosis, balanitis, or paraphimosis
- Low risk to get urinary tract infections
- Lower risk for sexually transmitted infections, including HIV
- Lower risk of cancer of the penis
- Female sex partner has lower risk of getting cervical cancer

After the circumcision, Vaseline is applied to the head of the penis, and a piece of gauze is wrapped around the penis. The circumcision heals in seven to ten days.

Call the doctor in case of the following:

- If there is persistent bleeding
- If there is redness or swelling of the penis
- If there is foul-smelling yellow or green discharge
- If there is no urine for eight hours after the circumcision
- If the plastic ring is still on the penis after two weeks

A baby should not have circumcision under these circumstances:

- If there is a medical problem

- If he is premature
- If someone has a bleeding disorder in the family
- If he has a physical problem with his penis that may need surgery later on like hypospadias or chordee. *Hypospadias* is a birth defect in which the opening of the penis is on the underside instead of the tip of the penis. *Chordee* is a curvature of the penis. Both conditions need surgery.

If your child is not circumcised, it is very important to keep the penis clean. In the first year, the foreskin does not retract. Do not force it back. Later you need to teach your child how to clean the penis.

Good to know

You can convert pounds (lbs) to kilogram (kg) by dividing pounds with 2.2

- 1 ounce = 30 grams
- 1 pint = 16 ounces
- 1 quart = 1 liter
- 1 pound = 16 ounces
- 1 milliliter (ml) = 1 cubic centimeter (1cc)
- 1 teaspoon = 5ml
- 1 tablespoon = 15 ml
- 1 yard = 1 meter = 3 feet = 36 inches
- 1 foot = 12 inches = 30 centimeter (cm)
- 1 inch = 2.5 cm

The way to give medications and/or fluids:

- p.o. means by mouth
- sublingual is under the tongue
- IV (intravenous) is through the vein
- IM is into the muscle
- SC is under the skin
- per rectum means into the rectum

Temperature conversion

- 96.8 degrees Fahrenheit (F) = 36 degrees Celsius (C)
- 97.8 degrees F = 36.6 degrees C
- 98.6 degrees F = 37.0 degrees C
- 99.4 degrees F = 37.4 degrees C
- 99.7 degrees F = 37.6 degrees C
- 100.1 degrees F = 37.8 degrees C
- 100.4 degrees F = 38 degrees C
- 101 degrees F = 38.3 degrees C

- 102.2 degrees F = 39 degrees C
- 102.6 degrees F = 39.2 degrees C
- 103.3 degrees F = 39.6 degrees C
- 104 degrees F = 40 degrees C
- 105 degrees F = 40.6 degrees C
- 105.8 degrees F = 41 degrees C

If your child's temperature is below 99.6 degrees F, he or she has no fever.

If your child's temperature is less than 100 degrees F, there is no need to give fever reducers like Tylenol or ibuprofen unless he or she has a history of seizures.

If your baby has a fever, see the doctor. But in the first two to three months, go to the emergency room.

When you give liquid medicine to your child, always use a measuring spoon, dropper, or syringe. Do not use a regular teaspoon or tablespoon.

Babies need to have at least four to six wet diapers over twenty-four hours.

Children need to urinate at least four times over twenty-four hours. If they have less than that, they need to drink more fluids.

If there is no urine for eight to nine hours, go to the emergency room.

Babies usually have more than one stool over twenty-four hours. And children need to have one bowel movement a day. Breastfed babies can have four to six stools a day and they can be loose. But they can also have stools only every three days.

Antibiotics do not cure viral illnesses. If they are overused, the germs develop resistance against them, and they do not work when we need them to cure bacterial infections.

The same way superbugs are created, and that means that no antibiotic is effective against them.

If your baby's milk is formula, no extra vitamins are needed unless ordered by the doctor. Formulas have the daily recommended vitamins.

Breastfed babies need vitamin D and iron supplement.

Milk is low in iron and vitamin D (unless fortified with vitamin D).

Iron and vitamin D supplement is needed as recommended by the doctor.

Honey cannot be given before one year of age because it can cause a severe disease called botulism.

Egg white cannot be given before one year of age because it can cause an allergic reaction.

Do not give regular milk to your baby before one year of age.

Do not give your child milk or milk-based formula if he or she vomited or had diarrhea.

Some dietary supplements can be harmful.

Incubation period is the time period between exposure to an infection and the appearance of the first symptoms.

An acute condition means that the symptoms appear suddenly and the disease has a short duration.

Chronic condition is one that develops slowly over a longer period of time and is long-lasting.

Pain rating scale

The intensity of pain can be assessed. If your child has pain, the doctor probably will ask, "How do you rate your pain on a scale of 1 to 10?"

- A rating from 1 to 3 is mild pain.
- A rating from 3 to 6 is moderate pain.
- A rating from 7 to 9 is severe pain.
- A rating of 10 is very severe pain.

Immunizations

Immunizations are very important to prevent serious infections.

There are some diseases when immunization is the only mean to fight a serious and often lethal disease.

Immunization is the process by which a person's immune system becomes protected against a bacteria or a virus. By the introduction of an agent (immunogen) unknown to the body, the immune system responds, fighting that agent. It will also remember that agent and will respond to it in a future encounter.

This method is called active immunization and is used universally.

The other method is called passive immunization. That means that we introduce antibodies to a sick child to fight a severe infection. The antibodies were developed by the immune system of another person who had the same infection.

Passive immunization is only used in selected cases.

Most vaccines are given by shot (inoculation).

Until the nineteenth century, there was no protection against serious infectious diseases. The first vaccine was developed against a deadly disease, smallpox.

Since then, several vaccines were made, mostly in the twentieth century.

Often, different vaccines are combined in order to give fewer shots to children.

Booster shots are given after the basic immunization series is done. That reminds the body's immune system of the infectious agent (immunogen) given by the shot. That way the body's immunity is enhanced, and the fighting capability against that specific infection is increased.

It is important to start the vaccines early on to protect the babies in a time when they are most vulnerable because their immune system is not fully developed.

The presently available and recommended vaccines for every child are summarized in the following **immunization schedule:**

Hepatitis B

- First dose at birth
- Second dose at one or two months of age
- Third dose six through eighteen months of age

Rotavirus vaccine

- Two and four months of age if Rotarix (RV1) is used
- Two, four, and six months if RotaTeq (RV5) is used

Rotavirus vaccine is given by mouth.

DTaP (diphtheria, tetanus, pertussis)

- Two, four, and six months
- Booster shot at fifteen through eighteen months, then four through six years

IPV (inactivated polio vaccine)

- IPV shot is given at ages two months, four months, and six to eighteen months
- Booster shot four through six years

HIB (Haemophilus influenzae type b)

- Two, four, and six months
- If PedvaxHIB is given, only two doses are needed at two and four months
- Booster shot at twelve through fifteen months

PCV 13 or PCV 15 or PCV 20 (pneumococcal vaccine)

- Two, four, and six months

- Booster shot at twelve through fifteen months

MMR (measles, mumps, rubella)

- Twelve through fifteen months
- Booster shot four through six years

VAR chickenpox (varicella)

- Twelve through fifteen months
- Booster shot four through six years

Hepatitis A

- Two doses at twelve through twenty-three months. The two doses are separated by six to eighteen months.

Meningococcal vaccine

- Menactra or Menveo eleven through twelve years old
- Booster shot at sixteen years old

Meningococcal B vaccine

- Bexsero or Trumenba is given to children who have high risk conditions or increased risk for the disease. Two doses are recommended, the second dose given at least six months after the first one.
- College students have a higher risk of meningitis caused by the bacteria meningococcus than other teenagers and young adults who are not attending college.

HPV (human papillomavirus)

- Eleven to twelve years old

- However, the first dose can be given after nine years of age
- After the first dose, the second dose is in one or two months, and the third dose is six months after the second dose

Other, not scheduled immunizations

Influenza vaccination is recommended for every child after six months of age and over, every year, before the "flu season" starts.

There is also an influenza vaccine that is a nasal spray—FluMist. It is sprayed into the nose.

Hepatitis A immune globulin is given within two weeks after exposure to hepatitis A. This is a passive immunization.

Immune globulin is given within six days of exposure to measles.

Varicella-zoster immune globulin (VZIG) can be given after exposure to chickenpox in selected cases.

Immune globulin decreases the efficacy of the vaccines; therefore, there should be an interval of five to eight months between the administration of immune globulin and a vaccine like measles, chickenpox, etc.

Children with high-risk conditions like chronic heart, lung, kidney disease, cancer, sickle cell disease have a decreased capability to fight infections (immunodeficiency). Therefore, they need pneumococcal vaccine—Pneumovax23-PPSV23—to protect against a germ called *streptococcus pneumoniae* (pneumococcus). This vaccine protects against twenty-three types of pneumococcal bacteria that cause pneumococcal diseases. Prevnar13 protects against thirteen types of pneumococcal bacteria.

Pneumovax 23 is given between two and five years of age.

Booster shot is needed five years after the first one.

Pneumovax 23 can only be given if the PCV 13 series is completed, and at least eight weeks after that. Children from two through eighteen years old with certain medical conditions should receive Pneumovax 23-PPSV23. RSV vaccine (Abrysvo) for pregnant women to protect the baby. RSV vaccines Synagis and nirsevimab for infants.

Newborns whose mother have hepatitis B receive hepatitis B immunoglobulin (passive immunization) and the first hepatitis B vaccine at birth.

Children with animal bite, scratch, open wound contaminated with saliva, when rabies is suspected, need human rabies vaccine and rabies immune globulin. The latter one is passive immunization (see above).

Typhoid vaccine is available for the prevention of typhoid fever (see diarrhea).

If a child needs tetanus shot after eight years of age, then Tdap or Td should be given instead of DTaP DT.

COVID-19 vaccine is available for children after six months of age.

Dengue vaccine (Dengvaxia) is available for the prevention of severe dengue disease. It is recommended for children aged nine to sixteen who have confirmation of previous dengue disease and lives in an area where dengue disease is common (epidemic). A previous dengue infection should be confirmed by lab test before the shot is given, otherwise the child can get a severe form of the disease if he gets the dengue virus after getting the shot.

Smallpox vaccine has not been given anymore because the disease is eradicated, and the vaccine can have serious side effects.

Combination vaccines:

- DTaP contains a combination of diphtheria, tetanus, and pertussis (whooping cough) vaccines.
- MMR is a combination of measles, mumps, and rubella (German measles) vaccines.
- MMRV is like MMR but also includes chickenpox vaccine (varicella). The name of the vaccine is ProQuad.
- DTaP-IPV-HepB, the name of the vaccine is Pediarix.
- DTaP-IPV-Hib, the name of the vaccine is Pentacel.
- DTaP- IPV, the name of the vaccine is Kinrix.
- DTaP-IPV-HIB-HepB, the name of the vaccine is Vaxelis.

- HepB-Hib, the name of the vaccine is Comvax.
- HepA-HepB is the combination of Hepatitis A and Hepatitis B vaccine. The name of the vaccine is Twinrix.
- Hib MenCY is the combination of HIB and meningococcal vaccine. The name of the vaccine is MenHibrix.

The immunization schedule directs the doctors to what age to give the vaccines.

Immunizations do not mean that the child will have 100 percent protection against the diseases he or she was immunized against. But after the vaccination, it is much less likely that the child will get the disease, and if he or she develops the disease, it is usually milder.

Parents and caregivers are recommended to have the Tdap vaccine if there is a newborn or a young baby in the house because adults can transfer whooping cough to babies even if they do not show symptoms or only have a mild cough.

Immunizations during pregnancy

Pregnant women are recommended to get flu shot but not FluMist because that is a live vaccine.

Get a Tdap (tetanus, diphtheria, pertussis) shot right after delivery. TdaP shot needs to be repeated with each pregnancy. This shot protects you and your baby from whooping cough (pertussis).

Immunizations not recommended during pregnancy:

- measles, mumps, and rubella
- human papillomavirus
- chickenpox (varicella)
- FluMist

Travel vaccines:

- typhoid fever (oral and injectable)
- yellow fever

- Japanese encephalitis

A vaccine should never be given again (contraindicated) if the child had a severe allergic reaction after a previous dose or is allergic to any component of the vaccine.

Call the doctor if you think your child has any side effects after the administration of a vaccine. However, if he has a severe allergic reaction, call 911 (see allergies: allergic reaction).

Children with decreased ability to fight infections (immune deficiency) should not have the following live vaccines:

- Rotavirus
- Live polio vaccine (OPV oral vaccine or Sabin vaccine given by mouth). Naturally they get the polio shot, the inactivated polio vaccine (IPV)
- MMR (measles, mumps, rubella)
- Varivax (chickenpox) or MMRV (measles, mumps, rubella, chickenpox)
- Flu Mist (LAIV- Live Attenuated Influenza Vaccine)
- Yellow Fever
- Oral typhoid vaccine
- BCG
- Smallpox

DTaP and Tdap should not be given again if the child had decreased level of consciousness, prolonged seizures, not attributable to any other identifiable cause and within seven days of administration of a previous dose.

Vaccines are temporarily withheld if the child has a moderate or severe illness or if he or she has tuberculosis.

The vaccines protect against the diseases below:

- Rotavirus causes diarrhea, often severe, that can lead to dehydration.

- Diphtheria is a bacterial disease that can cause upper airway obstruction and severe respiratory distress.
- Whooping cough (pertussis) is a bacterial disease causing severe cough. It is most serious for babies because they can stop breathing from it.
- Tetanus (lockjaw) is a bacterial disease. It is often lethal. It can develop from dirty wounds, causing painful muscle cramps, seizures, lockjaw. Meningitis can occur too (see vomiting).
- Haemophilus influenzae is a bacteria causing infection around the brain (meningitis), pneumonia, ear infections, severe bone, joint, and other infections.
- Pneumococcus is a bacteria causing infection around the brain (meningitis), pneumonia, and other often serious infections.
- Measles is a viral infection that can cause inflammation of the brain (encephalitis), pneumonia, and other illnesses.
- Mumps is a viral infection that can cause inflammation of the brain (encephalitis), a disease of the pancreas, also the testicles and ovaries (mostly in adolescents).
- Rubella is a viral disease that can rarely cause inflammation around the brain (encephalitis) and joint pain. The most severe problem caused by rubella occurs if the mother gets it during the first three months of pregnancy. The newborn can have severe anomalies of the eyes, heart, brain, and the liver and spleen can be enlarged. Hearing also can be affected.
- Chickenpox (varicella) is a viral disease that can cause skin infection and rarely inflammation of the brain (encephalitis), kidney, and liver problems. Fortunately, severe side effects caused by measles, mumps, rubella, and chickenpox are rare.
- Meningococcus is a bacteria causing infection around the brain (meningitis), other infections, and shock.

- Hepatitis A is a viral disease causing inflammation of the liver.
- Hepatitis B is a viral disease causing inflammation of the liver. Hepatitis B can be transmitted from the mother to the newborn baby.
- Human papillomavirus can cause genital warts and development of cervical cancer.
- Influenza is a viral disease that can cause pneumonia, ear infection, and other diseases.
- Rabies is a viral disease. It causes infection around the brain (encephalitis), and it is usually lethal.
- Dengue fever is caused by a viral infection and is transmitted by mosquitoes. It can cause severe disease with respiratory distress, bleeding, and organ damage.
- RSV is a viral disease, causing respiratory symptoms, often bronchiolitis (see bronchiolitis), that can cause problem breathing. Premature babies are especially vulnerable to RSV infection.

All of the above diseases are contagious with the exception of tetanus, rabies, and dengue fever
(see infectious diseases of childhood).

Misconceptions

1. False: teething can cause fever. True: Teething might increase the temperature by a few tenth of a degree of Fahrenheit. However, if the child has high fever, it will be a different cause.
2. False: the more milk a child drinks, the healthier he or she will be. True: It is true that milk is healthy, but large amounts can take the child's appetite away and can cause anemia that can be severe.
3. False: the more vitamins a child takes, the healthier he or she will be. True: vitamins are important, but too much may be harmful.
4. False: if the mother takes vitamins and breastfeeds, the baby does not need vitamins. True: The amount of vitamins, particularly vitamin D, that the baby gets from breast milk is not sufficient. The baby needs to take his or her own vitamins, as recommended by the doctor.
5. False: walkers help babies to walk sooner. True: The child will walk when he or she is ready, regardless. Besides, walkers can tip over, causing injury.
6. False: when a child has a cold, he or she needs Tylenol. True: The child only needs Tylenol if he has fever or pain.
7. False: if a child has an infection, he needs antibiotics. True: That is only true if the child has a bacterial infection. Antibiotics do not work against viral infections, and if overused, the germs get stronger, and the antibiotic will not work when needed.
8. False: marijuana use is not harmful. True: marijuana causes fast heart rate, impaired abstract thinking, and driving ability. Overdose causes anxiety. Regular use of marijuana can lead to mental and lung problems.
9. False: if the child has no fever, he is not sick. True: other symptoms like vomiting, lethargy are even more important.

Sex education

Sexuality education includes teaching about human sexuality, intimate relationships, sexual anatomy, sexual reproduction, sexual activity, abstinence, contraception, sexual orientation, gender identity, sexually transmitted diseases (STD), and sexual responsibilities.

It is important to provide developmentally appropriate, evidence-based, and medically correct information.

Parents, schools, pediatricians, and other health professionals can give that information.

Your child's doctor can be a good source. He or she can discuss issues with you and your child together and separately. Assurance of confidentiality is important.

LGBT youth should be included in sex education.

While abstinence is the best way to avoid teen pregnancies and sexually transmitted diseases, the use of condom with each sexual encounter is most important.

A girl who is sexually active needs to see a gynecologist, and he or she can give her advice on contraception.

Sports physicals

Sport and exercise are beneficial for all children and adolescents. But yearly preparticipation physical exam is necessary and required for organized sports.

The doctor takes a history, including family history, and does a physical exam.

If any heart problem is suspected, additional tests are done like ECG and echocardiogram.

Sometimes a referral is needed to a pediatric cardiologist.

Children with known heart disease can usually do some sports and exercises as recommended by their cardiologist.

However, there are some diseases when playing sports can be dangerous and therefore contraindicated.

If a child, for example, has a so-called hypertrophic cardiomyopathy (see heart problems), he cannot participate in sports. This disease is usually inherited, so tell the doctor if anybody has it in your family.

Toilet training

Toilet training usually starts after two years of age. But some children are not ready before age three, since the maturation of the nervous system and muscles of the bladder varies from child to child. Some children continue wetting the bed until age five. There is no rush, because if you start too early, it might take longer to train your child. You will have some idea when your child is ready for toilet training. When he will feel that a bowel movement is coming, he will make a certain face or noise or move into a corner. He might also show interest in urine or stool. When your child seems to be ready for training, show him the connection between the stool and the potty. You can point out stool and show it as it is flushed down the toilet. Let him do it. When you see that your child will have a bowel movement, place him on the potty. Encourage your child to stay on the potty, and if there is success, praise him happily. Even if your child only sits on the potty without result, praise him for trying. Be patient. Never press or criticize him, and show no frustration, because that can push back the process of toilet training. Even if your child is toilet-trained, accidents still can happen. Do not scold, shame, or discipline him. If your child resists, do not fight, but stop the training for a while and start again. Do not hurry to change the diapers to training pants or underwear. Wait a couple of weeks of successful potty training. Celebrate the transition.

Nighttime and nap time training takes longer. Most children stay dry at five to seven years of age.

Teach your child, particularly your daughter, to always wipe from front to back to prevent germs from getting to the urethra, causing urinary tract infection.

Teach your child early on to wash his hands after using the potty or toilet.

If you have problems with potty training, call the doctor.

2

The Not-So-Well Child

The largest part of this book talks about some diseases children can get. I want you to be prepared to recognize them and know what to do. However, fortunately, children are healthy most of the time.

Acne

Acne may appear in the neonatal period. Newborn acne resolves spontaneously. In adolescence, blackheads, whiteheads, and pimples can be seen. Acne is most often located on the face, and on the back. They can get infected. In that case, the pimples get red and have pus (pustules).

The most severe form is when cyst develops. Scarring also occurs.

Treatment

Local treatment often starts with benzoyl peroxide. If an infection is present, antibiotics are given. Severe acne can be treated with a vitamin A derivative given by mouth such as Accutane. This medication can cause severe side effects and is contraindicated during pregnancy. It should not be taken with vitamin A and tetracycline. If the acne is severe, usually a skin doctor (dermatologist) is involved in the care of the child. It is important to treat acne to prevent scarring.

Allergies: allergic reaction

Allergy is an increased sensitivity and response of the body to specific substances, called allergens. The fact that one has not had an allergy in the past is not a guarantee for the future. Many things can cause allergies, like medications, foods, insect bites and inhaled allergens.

Any medication can cause an allergic problem, but most commonly antibiotics. Food allergies are most commonly caused by nuts (most commonly peanuts), eggs, cow milk, shellfish, fish, less commonly wheat and soy. Insect bites most often causing allergic reactions are ants, bees, wasps, hornets.

Children, just as adults, can develop allergies at any age. It is more likely that the child develops allergies if one or both parents have them.

A baby can have an *allergy to cow's milk*. Symptoms are vomiting, diarrhea (sometimes bloody), and abdominal cramps. Rarely an allergic rash develops. A baby who is allergic to cow's milk formula is usually switched to soy formula. But he or she can be allergic to that too, and in that case, the next option is elemental formula (amino acid hydrolysate), like Nutramigen or Alimentum.

Hay fever (*allergic rhinitis*) is a common allergy. Symptoms are stuffy nose and watery itchy eyes. But frequent sneezing, rubbing of the nose because of itching (allergic salute), and dark circles around the eyes are also common.

In the beginning, it is hard to distinguish an allergic nasal congestion from a "cold" (upper respiratory infection). But in the case of an allergy, the mucus remains clear, while in the case of a cold, the color of the mucus turns to yellow, then green, and clear again. Also, the duration is different. If it is an allergy, it lasts much longer and often recurs. The recurrence can happen in certain seasons. The symptoms also can be present all year around.

Allergies can cause pink eye (*allergic or vernal conjunctivitis*).

Symptoms are itchy eyes, redness, watery discharge, swelling of the conjunctiva (the tissue covering the white part of the eye and the inner surface of the eyelid), and often sensitivity to light.

Asthma is a severe allergic response to allergens at the lower respiratory tract and is characterized by cough and often trouble breathing.

Nasal allergy and asthma are usually caused by inhaled allergens like dust, house dust mites, molds, and cockroaches, ragweed, etc.

Asthma symptoms are coughing spells, wheezing, often respiratory problems (see cough, respiratory problems, respiratory distress).

Hives and eczema–atopic dermatitis are common skin manifestations of allergies. Hives are raised pink areas on the skin. Eczema symptoms are red itchy and irritated skin. Scratching the itchy skin can lead to infection. Belts that contain nickel can cause skin irritation (*contact dermatitis*). Nickel allergy also can be associated with earrings.

Allergic reaction

A child who has allergies can develop an allergic reaction.

Symptoms are rash, slightly raised pink areas (hives), itching, swelling of the eyelids, lips, hands and feet.

The swelling can develop at one or more parts of the body.

An allergic reaction can be severe, causing symptoms of croup, asthma, and it can lead to shock.

The croup-like symptoms are barking cough and audible raspy breathing. The child may have difficulty with inhalation secondary to upper airway obstruction. If it is severe, there is pulling in under the Adam's apple in front of the neck (see cough, respiratory problems, respiratory distress).

Asthma symptoms are coughing spells, wheezing, and often respiratory problems (see cough, respiratory problems, respiratory distress).

Asthma symptoms can be severe. The child can have difficulty breathing, and pulling in can be seen under the rib cage.

If shock develops, the symptoms are dizziness, change in consciousness, fast heart rate, and breathing.

The hands and feet will be cold. The skin can be mottled and bluish. If you press the finger or toenails, the color will not return to normal within two seconds as it normally does (slow capillary refill). Vomiting and diarrhea can be present as well, and cold sweat.

All three conditions—croup, asthma, and shock—can cause color change. The child can be extremely pale or have a blue discoloration of the lips, face, fingernails.

In case of an allergic reaction, urgent medical attention is necessary.

Go to the emergency room or call 911. But in case of labored breathing, color change, and altered consciousness, call 911.

A severe allergic reaction is called anaphylaxis. Treatment of allergies: drugs like Benadryl, Claritin, Zyrtec, Allegra (antihistamines) work for hay fever.

Avoidance diet. Avoid foods that the child is allergic to. Do not give him or her foods that often cause allergies. Be sure your child never takes medicine that caused an allergic reaction in the past.

Treatment of nasal allergies (allergic rhinitis): Saline nasal spray to clear the nostrils, and get rid of the allergens. But the most effective treatment is a steroid nasal spray.

Treatment of allergic conjunctivitis (pink eye): antihistamine eye drops, like Patanol, Pataday, and Zaditor.

Treatment of eczema: Use a mild soap, like Aveeno, Dove, Neutrogena. Use a moisturizer cream, like Eucerin, Aquaphor, Cetaphil after bathing. Steroid ointment if needed. In case of severe eczema, a skin doctor (dermatologist) is often consulted.

Treatment of asthma: Medications like Albuterol to open up the airways (bronchodilators). They are usually delivered by a so-called nebulizer or inhaler (see cough, respiratory problems, respiratory distress). Steroids. They can be given by injection, by mouth, or by a nebulizer or inhaler.

In case of severe allergies and asthma, a lung doctor (pulmonologist) or allergist often participates in the child's care.

Sometimes so-called immunotherapy is used. Small amounts of the antigen is given to the child with injections about once a week, and the dose is gradually increased so the body can get used to the allergen. The treatment can last for years.

Treatment of allergic reaction: epinephrine shot, antihistamine, steroid

If your child has an allergic reaction, and you have epinephrine (EpiPen) with you, give your child a dose.

If you have Benadryl or any other antihistamine, give your child a dose, unless he or she vomits or has a change in consciousness. But **give the EpiPen first**. After that, go to the emergency room or call 911.

If there is louder, harder breathing, color change, swelling of the tongue or neck, if he feels that his throat is closing, or there is a change of consciousness, call 911.

To prevent another allergic reaction, again, be sure that your child never takes the medicine or food that caused the allergic reaction in the first place. Also, if your child had an allergic reaction from a medicine, tell the doctor every time that he or she is allergic to that medicine.

If your child has had an allergic reaction, it is necessary to carry epinephrine (EpiPen) all the time, just in case. The school and camp also needs to have it as well.

For nasal allergy and asthma, it can make a difference if you take old rugs, curtains, and stuffed animals out of your child's room because they retain the dust. A good steam cleaning of the carpet also can help. Hardwood floors are preferable to carpet. Remove dust with a wet cloth. Encase the pillows and mattresses with plastic covering. Change the air conditioner filters regularly and use high efficiency air filters. If the child has asthma, cigarette smoke, including secondhand smoke, is particularly harmful. Pet animals are best kept outside. Buy goldfish.

If you suspect that your child has an allergy problem, see the doctor.

Altitude sickness

At high altitude, 8,000 feet (2,500 meters), the air has less oxygen, and that can cause symptoms of altitude sickness, also called acute mountain sickness. Altitude sickness can be mild but can be dangerous as well. Rapid ascent to high altitude is a risk.

Symptoms are headache, decreased appetite, nausea, vomiting, feeling weak, dizzy, and having trouble sleeping.

Altitude sickness is dangerous, even life-threatening when it affects the brain or the lungs. If the child is confused, cannot walk straight, feeling faint, having problem breathing, or having a bluish color of the lips, around the lips, and fingernails, urgent medical attention is needed, and take your child to a lower altitude right away. If your child develops warning signs like severe headache, nausea, or problem with coordination, it is time to descend.

To prevent altitude sickness, go slowly, and gradually ascend to higher places. Rest much and take plenty of fluids. It is recommended to avoid high altitudes with babies under one year of age and young children since they are more susceptible to severe high altitude sickness.

Prepare for cold temperatures. Before you go to a place with high altitude, check out first how many feet high it is. Be sure your child is in good physical shape before going to places with high altitude. Children with preexisting medical problems should consult with the doctor before the trip.

Anemia (paleness)

If a baby or a child looks pale, there is a suspicion that he is anemic.

Anemia means that the number of red blood cells are diminished and the concentration of the hemoglobin in the red blood cells is decreased. The hemoglobin binds the oxygen molecules, providing oxygen to the body.

Babies normally have some gradual decrease of red blood cells and hemoglobin between two to three months of age. It is called *physiologic anemia.*

There are different types of anemias. The most common one is *iron deficiency anemia,* caused by insufficient iron intake.

Infants who are breastfed need iron supplements because breast milk is low in iron. The iron is usually provided by multivitamins with iron. The baby needs to take these drops daily. Even if the mother takes vitamins, the amount getting to the breast milk is not sufficient. Discuss it with the doctor.

Premature and low birth weight babies are more susceptible to iron deficiency.

Too much milk intake also can cause iron deficiency anemia, and it can be severe. Cow's milk is low in iron, and if a child drinks too much of it, he or she will not eat enough solids that would provide iron. Also, too much milk can cause small bleeding in the gut. Therefore, it is not recommended to give more cow's milk to a child than sixteen ounces per day.

Babies should not drink more milk-based formula than thirty-two ounces per day.

Iron-fortified formulas provide a sufficient amount of iron. However, breastfeeding is still far superior. Breast milk has the optimal formulation and immunoglobulins to fight infections.

The introduction of solids, iron fortified cereals, vegetables, fruits, then meat to the infant's diet provide some iron. After infancy, a healthy diet can give the child a sufficient amount of iron.

Some foods that are rich in iron are liver, red meat, cream of wheat, spinach, prune, raisin, navy bean.

If your child is pale, has a poor appetite, or wants to eat unusual things like dirt, visit the doctor, because these symptoms can be caused by iron deficiency anemia.

The diagnosis is made by blood test.

If the iron level is low, the child needs iron supplementation or iron therapy.

Other causes of anemia

Elevated lead level. If you live in a house built before 1978, when homes were painted with lead-based paint, let the doctor know.

Bleeding. It can be acute bleeding from an injury or can be chronic bleeding, when small amounts of blood loss persist for a long time. The origin is most often the gut.

Destruction of the red blood cells (hemolytic anemia), chronic infection, inflammation, abnormal hemoglobin, as in sickle cell anemia or thalassemia, decreased red blood cell production of the bone marrow, enzyme defects, and abnormally shaped red blood cells (spherocytosis) also can cause anemia (see below).

Sickle cell disease. Sickle cell anemia is an inherited hemoglobin anomaly. It is most common in African American children.

Symptoms include fatigue, paleness, jaundice. Fever, headache, pain in the extremities (often severe), enlargement of the spleen, liver, or heart can occur.

The child is more susceptible to severe bacterial infections.

Children with sickle cell anemia can have very severe pain secondary to the so-called sickle cell crisis. The child also can have aplastic crisis, when the red blood cell production is diminished on top of the ongoing red blood cell destruction.

Since the red blood cells transport oxygen to the different organs of the body, severe anemia can cause heart failure, breathing problems, and shock.

The diagnosis is made by blood test.

Treatment:

- Fluids
- Painkillers
- Antibiotics if infection is suspected
- Hydroxyurea
- Severe anemia is treated with transfusion

For the prevention of severe bacterial infections, penicillin is given regularly. Immunization with pneumococcal vaccine (PCV) is extremely important.

Thalassemia. Thalassemia is a hemoglobin defect. It has different forms. Because of the destruction of red blood cells, severe anemia can develop.

If a child does not have the disease but the thalassemia trait, he or she still can be anemic, but to a lesser degree. The diagnosis is made by hemoglobin analysis. Treatment in severe cases is transfusion.

Congenital (hereditary) spherocytosis. This disease is inherited. The red blood cells are abnormally shaped, they get excessively destroyed, leading to anemia that can be severe.

The diagnosis is made by blood test. Treatment is removal of the spleen (splenectomy).

Deficiency of vitamin B_{12} and folate deficiency also can cause anemia, namely, pernicious anemia or macrocytic megaloblastic anemia. The treatment is vitamin supplement (see vitamins).

If a child has any of these diseases, he usually needs to see a hematologist.

Appetite, poor appetite, overeating

Appetite is an instinct. So if a baby is healthy, he or she should have a good appetite.

The appetite is poor only if there is a problem (disease or disorder) or if the baby or child has developed bad eating habits with the help of adults.

Parents commonly complain that their child eats very little.

However, when the weight is checked, it is perfectly normal. It is not easy to judge how much food a baby or child needs and how much is too little or too much. Even when there are siblings, a comparison is maybe not correct because different children eat different amounts of food. The important thing is that the child has good weight gain and his or her weight is in the normal range and appropriate for the height when checked on the growth chart.

How do bad feeding habits develop? If the baby is fed every time he or she cries or starts to cry. If we let an older baby or toddler pick up the milk bottle whenever he or she wants it. If we give the child milk or juice all the time or every time he or she prefers it over a regular meal.

The same is true about snacks. If we give the child too much milk, juice, snacks, there will be no appetite left for regular meals. Besides, drinking too much milk can cause anemia (see anemia).

On-demand feeding does not mean that the baby can eat all the time, for example every hour. Very frequent feedings can cause vomiting too.

Do not push your child to eat because that develops opposition, and the child will refuse the food. Force-feeding is an absolute no-no.

The condition when a child does not gain weight appropriately or his or her weight lags behind is called failure to thrive (FTT) (see failure to thrive).

Older children often prefer junk food. That should be limited.

Overeating

Eating all the time can cause obesity.

Do not push your baby to finish the bottle, or your child to finish all the food that is in front of him or her, because it can become a habit and leads to obesity.

Babies do not need desserts. You do not want your baby to be overweight. If a baby or toddler is overweight, there is a good chance that he or she will be overweight as an adult.

Children often want to drink sweet drinks, sodas. That gives them extra sugar, extra calories they do not need, and can be harmful. Drinking water instead should be encouraged.

Watching TV or playing video games for a long time and eating during that time, particularly sweets, is a common cause of getting overweight. It is okay to say no to your child.

Athlete's foot

Athlete's foot is a fungal disease.

The skin becomes reddish on the toes, between the toes, and often on the sole. Peeling and cracking of the skin is common. There is itching, but there also can be pain because of the cracks.

Prevention: Have your child wear flip-flops at public pools and showers. After a bath or shower, be sure that he thoroughly dries his feet, paying particular attention to the toes and the skin in between toes. Do not let your child wear rubber or plastic shoes without socks. The best practice is to wear cotton socks and change them daily.

Treatment is antifungal cream or powder. If there is no improvement in a week or two, see the doctor.

Back pain

Injuries can cause back pain. If it is serious, lay the child down on the ground, and do not move him or her, and **call 911**.

Back pain is more common in adolescents, particularly if they play sports. Back pain in a young child is more worrisome.

If a child has back pain for more than a few days, he or she needs to see the doctor.

Important questions:

- Is there any history of trauma?
- When did the pain start?
- Does it radiate anywhere?
- What part of the back hurts?
- How strong is the pain? Does it wake the child up at night?
- Is the pain permanent or recurring? If it is recurring pain, how frequent is it?
- Does the child play sports? If the answer is yes, what sport does he or she play, and how intensive is the sport?
- Does the child have a heavy backpack?
- Is there any deformity?
- Does the child have fever, malaise, weight loss, or any other symptoms?
- Is there any limitation of movements? Can he walk well?
- Is there any muscle weakness or tingling?
- Does the child have any systemic disease?
- Is there any problem holding the urine or stool?
- Is the urination okay?

Causes of back pain:

- Bad posture, a heavy backpack, obesity.
- A child can have muscle strain, particularly after playing sports or lifting weights.

- Girls can have back pain around the time they have their period.
- Abdominal pain can radiate to the back in case of gallbladder disease.
- If the child has influenza, body ache is common, and that includes back pain.
- Lower back pain can be caused by kidney diseases.
- Structural problems and diseases of the spine cause back pain.

Some of these structural problems and diseases:

- Curvature of the spine (scoliosis) (see flat foot and other orthopedic problems).
- Hunchback (Scheuermann) disease (see flat foot and other orthopedic problems).
- That is a deformity of the spine. Even when the child leans backward, the appearance of the back does not change, and a hump can be seen.
- Treatment is brace or cast.
- Stress fracture of the spine (spondylolysis) and slippage of the vertebra (spondylolisthesis).
- Symptoms: The main symptom is back pain. Weakness, numbness of the legs can occur.
- X-ray, magnetic resonance imaging (MRI), and bone scan are often used to make the diagnosis.
- Treatment: limitation of physical activity and physical therapy.
- Rheumatic diseases like juvenile arthritis (see joint pain with systemic disease).

- Ankylosing spondylitis
  Stiffness of the back and back pain are characteristic.
- Tumors

Back pain and weakness of the lower extremities are frequent symptoms.
Treatment is usually surgery.
For all of the above diseases, orthopedic surgeons are participating in the child's care.

- Rarely, infection of the disc (flat plate between the vertebrae) can cause back pain.
The child keeps the spine straight, stiff, and does not want to bend over.
Treatment is antibiotics. Orthopedic consult is needed.

- Herniated disc (herniated nucleus pulposus [HNP])
It rarely occurs in childhood. If it occurs, it is in late adolescence. The soft center of the spinal disc (nucleus pulposus) pushes through a crack on the disc. It can irritate a nerve, and that can cause pain, numbness, and weakness in the arm or leg. Orthopedic surgeons treat this condition.
Treatment: medication, physical therapy, and if necessary, surgery.

Bad breath (halitosis)

Frequent causes are the following:

- tooth and gum problems
- infection of the tonsils and/or adenoids
- sinus infection
- hand, foot and mouth disease
- vomiting
- dehydration (often, acetone smell can be noticed in the breath)

Treatment:

- cure the underlying condition
- mouthwash
- regular toothbrushing
- flossing

Bed-wetting (enuresis)

Toilet training usually starts after two years of age. But some children are not ready before age three since the maturation of the nervous system and muscles of the bladder varies from child to child.

A child is a bedwetter if he or she wets the bed after five years of age (enuresis nocturna). But some children not only wet the bed at night but also wet their pants during the day (enuresis diurna).

Sometimes wetting of the bed and pants plus soiling of the pants occur together. More boys than girls have a problem with bedwetting.

Some children never had a dry night. Others were fully trained and then bedwetting returned. Also, some children wet the bed every night, others from time to time, while others again only occasionally.

Important questions:

- How old was the child when the toilet training was started?
- Was it easy or difficult? How did you do it? How did you act? Was there any discipline involved?
- Has the child ever been completely trained (not having accidents at all)?
- How often does bedwetting occur? Is it always about the same time?
- Is bedwetting a new phenomenon for her?
- Do the accidents occur only at night, or during the day too? Is there any soiling of the pants?
- Are there any complaints of urination?
- Is there a good strong urine stream?
- Are the bowel movements normal and regular?
- Does he drink and urinate as much as usual?
- Is there any change in your child's life?
- Does he or she have emotional problems?
- Is there any family problem?
- Is there any family member who used to have accidents, and what age did it stop?

Bedwetting can be "normal" if the child has no underlying physical or mental condition. Some children need more time to develop bladder control.

If a child has bedwetting, it is important to have a checkup to rule out any underlying condition and sort out possible causes.

Causes of enuresis:

- Delay of maturation
- Too early toilet training that was started before the child was ready
- Harsh toilet training
- Emotional problems
- Physical and mental conditions less commonly cause bed wetting, but they need to be ruled out

Physical diseases causing bedwetting are the following:

- Lower spinal cord lesions, including spina bifida (defective closure of the spine)
- Congenital anomalies of the urinary tract
- Urinary tract infections
- Kidney failure
- Chronic constipation
- Diabetes mellitus (commonly known as diabetes). The child drinks and urinates a lot because of the insufficient amount of insulin produced by the pancreas. The blood sugar is high (see thirst, drinking large amounts of fluids, and urinating a lot). Often, the first sign of diabetes is bed-wetting of a child who has not had accidents before.
- Diabetes insipidus. The pituitary gland does not produce enough antidiuretic hormone or vasopressin (ADH). That hormone is responsible for the conservation of water in the body. Also there is a condition when the kidneys do not respond to the ADH hormone. The result is thirst and

much urine production (see thirst, drinking large amounts of fluids, and urinating a lot).

Treatment of bed-wetting:

- The first rule is not to scorn or discipline your child for accidents. Do not show frustration or disappointment when you need to change the bed.
- Reassure your child that this is only a temporary condition that will be resolved over time.
- Let your child know if a relative had the same problem and what age it disappeared (it is common that other relatives have enuresis in the same family).
- Praise your child for every little success. Reward him or her for every dry night with a sticker or a star. Certain numbers of stickers or stars can add up for a bigger reward, like a small toy, movie ticket, or chocolate. It should not be too easy or too hard to get the present, and it should go along with praise when you give the sticker or a star (this method is called behavior modification).
- The most important thing is to get the child's cooperation and the will to succeed.
- Do not give much fluid to your child in the evening; rather, give it in the afternoon.
- Be sure that your child goes to the bathroom before going to bed.
- If the child always wets the bed about the same time, you can try to wake him or her up before that time every night for a while.
- If there are emotional problems, the child probably needs to see a psychologist. Emotional causes being the problem is more likely if the child wets during the day too, or soils his pants.
- The use of an alarm bell often helps. In that device, the alarm wakes up the child after the first few drops of urine

touches the pad. In case of relapse, the device can be used again.

- Medications also can be used. Imipramine but lately DDAVP has been used. DDAVP (vasopressin) is the hormone that reabsorbs the water from the kidneys. It has a high success rate but is only used after six years of age or if other non-pharmacological methods have not worked.

Behavioral problems and habits

Behavior problems

Attention deficit hyperactivity disorder (ADHD), attention deficit disorder (ADD). Since children are usually active, sometimes too active, parents often think they have ADHD. However, it is hard to make the diagnosis of ADHD before six years of age.

Usually, teachers bring up the likelihood of this condition. Questionnaires can help to make the diagnosis.

Important questions:

- Is your child hyper? Is he or she always on the move?
- Is your child restless? Squirmy?
- Is your child getting into everything?
- Is your child easily distracted?
- Does your child have problems focusing?
- Does your child have problems following instructions?
- Can your child stay on task and finish it?
- Is your child forgetful in daily activities?

A child can have attention deficit disorder without hyperactivity (ADD).

Psychologists are often helpful, particularly if the child has other symptoms as well.

Treatment: The child needs to be in a well-structured classroom with a small class. He or she needs to sit in the front of the class and needs more attention from teachers and also from parents to complete homework.

Stimulant medications like methylphenidate (Ritalin) or Adderall are used mostly to treat this condition.

Anxiety, anxiety disorder. Anxiety is a disproportionate fear of things, events, and situations. Anxiety can culminate in a panic attack. If a child is worried most of the time, he or she may have anxiety disorder. The child can worry about diseases, going to bed, and that the parents might get hurt. It can also be a problem separating from the parents or caretaker (*separation anxiety*) or a fear of going to school (*school phobia*).

Panic attack (*anxiety attack*). In that case, the child is terrified, sweating, and the heart rate and breathing are fast. The child takes fast and deep breaths (*hyperventilation*) and can pass out. Try to catch him if falling.

Treatment: If the child has significant and/or permanent anxiety, the doctor needs to be consulted.

The child might need to see a psychologist or psychiatrist.

If the child has an anxiety attack with fast and deep breathing, a plastic or brown bag should be placed over the nose and mouth, so the child will breathe in and out of the bag to prevent the loss of consciousness. When the child exhales, he blows out carbon dioxide. Loss of carbon dioxide is the problem. Breathing into the bag preserves carbon dioxide.

Temper tantrum. Toddlers can get upset easily when they want something and the parents say no.

They cry, scream, throw themselves down on the floor, and kick. This event can be embarrassing to the parents, particularly if it happens in a public place. They tend to give in to the child's demands, and that teaches the child that this behavior helps him to get what he wants.

Some toddlers cry so hard that they cannot catch their breath (*breath-holding spell*).

Their faces turn bluish, and they can pass out. Parents get frightened, but the condition is not dangerous. The only thing parents need to do is to prevent injury when the child falls down to the ground.

If your child has a temper tantrum, try to distract or ignore him or her.

If the child has breath-holding spells, he or she needs to see the doctor to be sure that the loss of consciousness is not secondary to a different condition, like seizure.

If temper tantrums occur after four years of age, probably a consultation with a psychologist is warranted.

Obsessive compulsive disorder (OCD). The characteristics are recurrent impulses, repetitive thoughts, rituals, and movements.

In times of stress, the child with OCD needs reassurance by doing the same thing over and over again. Constant handwashing, touching the same thing, checking the locks are common.

Treatment is psychotherapy and, if needed, medication.

Phobias. Many children have fears. Fear of dogs, strangers, separation from parents, and being alone in the dark are very common. But when the fear is out of proportion, unfounded, irrational, or inappropriate for the child's age, that is a phobia.

School phobia is important because the child does not want to go to school.

A child with an overanxious disorder has unrealistic worries about future events. He or she can have physical symptoms as well.

Treatment of phobias is behavioral therapy by a psychologist.

Oppositional defiant disorder (ODD). Continuous arguing, constant defiance of the rules. The child is resentful, spiteful, using obscene language. Aggression, antisocial behavior, delinquency can be present.

Conduct disorder. Lying, stealing, setting fire, cruelty to animals are the symptoms.

Depression

Important questions:

- Is your child always sad?
- How does your child sleep? Does he have a sleeping problem?

- Does your child have friends? If the answer is yes, does he or she hang out with them or play with them?
- Is your child interested in doing things that he or she always liked to do?
- Does your child play sports? If the answer is yes, does he or she play that sport at the present?
- Has your child said that life has no meaning?
- Has your child said "I wish I was dead"?
- Has your child said that he or she wants to hurt him or herself?
- Has your child hurt him or herself?

If the answer for most of these questions is yes, your child is probably depressed, and he or she needs to see the doctor, who will probably refer him or her to a psychiatrist. If there is any suicidal ideation or intentional injury, you have to take him or her to the emergency room or call 911 at once.

Telephone number for suicide prevention: Suicide and Crises Lifeline: 988.

Autism spectrum disorder (ASD). Autism is a complex developmental disability.

Important questions:

- Does your child like when you play with him or her?
- Does your child take an interest in other children?
- Does your child enjoy playing peekaboo?
- Does your child ever bring objects over to you to show you?
- Does your child look you in the eye for more than a second or two?
- Does your child smile in response to your face or smile?
- Does your child try to attract your attention to his or her activity?
- Does your child respond when you call his or her name?

- Does your child point with one finger to show you something?
- Does your child enjoy being swung or bounced on your knee?

If the answer for these questions is no, autism is suspected.

- Do you think your child has hearing problem?
- Does he have problem with speech?
- Does he repeat the same words over and over again?
- Does he have problem being touched?
- Does he like to be alone doing his own things and ignoring others?
- Does he have problem relating to others?
- Is your child very sensitive and gets upset at regular noises?
- Does your child make unusual finger movements near the eyes?
- Does your child sometimes stare at nothing or wonder with no purpose?

If the answer for these questions is yes, autism is suspected.

A child who has autism is not interested in communicating or playing with others. He or she plays alone, doing his own thing. What he or she is doing can be very meticulous.

Children who have autism often have speech problems.

Autism spectrum disorder can be mild or very severe.

Early recognition and treatment is important. Screenings are done at the checkups at eighteen and twenty-four months.

The goal is to improve speech, learning, behavior, and social skills. Treatment is special education, speech therapy, and applied behavioral analysis (ABA) of autism is an intensive treatment program. Occupational therapy (OT) and physical therapy (PT) are used as needed.

A milder form of autism is called *Asperger syndrome.*

This developmental disorder is on the higher functioning end of the autism spectrum. They have difficulty interacting socially but can be highly intelligent.

Habits

Thumb-sucking. Thumb-sucking is very common. It usually starts in infancy and stops at four to six years of age. It is a soothing activity that gives comfort to the child. If the habit is strong and lasts longer than expected, be sure not to embarrass the child. If thumb-sucking seems to be caused by emotional problems or stress, talk to the pediatrician. If the habit continues even after your child starts school, see the dentist. It needs to be checked whether it has resulted in misalignment of the teeth.

Nail-biting. Nail-biting is a habit that is not uncommon. The child can bite his nail if he is bored, anxious, or nervous. Nail-biting can cause skin infection on the finger.

What to do about nail biting?

- Trim the nails.
- Watch your child to see what triggers the nail-biting.
- Try to distract and comfort him.
- Praise him for not biting.
- Positive reinforcement and rewards can work. If he does not bite his nail for a certain amount of time, you give him a sticker. Certain amount of sticker means that he will have a small present, something that he likes. It should not be too easy or too hard to get the stickers and the present.

Head banging and rocking. These are rhythmic activities that soothe the baby or toddler. It can be normal but also can be related to developmental problems.

If the child has not stopped the habit by three years of age, or there are signs of a developmental problem, talk to the pediatrician.

Teeth grinding (bruxism). Grinding or clenching the teeth is more frequent at night. It can be secondary to misaligned teeth (mal-occlusion) or stress. In severe cases, the teeth can be affected; therefore, you want to see a dentist. A mouth guard may be fitted by the dentist.

Other habits. Some children have the habit of chewing things. Others play with their hair and pull it, causing hair loss (see hair loss). Another important habit is tic (see jerking and strange movements).

Treatment of habits: First of all, you want to divert your child's attention to something else. You want him or her to do something interesting, engaging, or his or her favorite activity.

You also can use positive reinforcement. You tell your child that if he or she stops doing the habit for a certain time, like an hour or two, you give him a star or small sticker, and put it in a notebook. Certain number of stars add up to a small present that your child likes. The task should not be too easy or too hard.

Birthmarks

Birthmarks are usually present at birth, but they can appear later as well. Birthmarks can be found anywhere on the skin, but some of them occur more often in certain locations.

For example, the so-called Mongolian spots are often seen on the shoulders, lower back, and buttocks.

Birthmarks can be vascular or pigmented in nature.

Vascular birthmarks. They are formed from blood vessels.

Stork bites. Many babies have so-called stork bites. Those are pink spots, frequently located on the forehead, eyelids, and on the back of the head (occiput). Stork bites are harmless and usually disappear with time.

Hemangiomas. The so-called strawberry hemangiomas are red masses of different sizes. They are made up of extra blood vessels in the skin. They can grow rapidly in the first few months but usually resolve spontaneously by the first year, sometimes leaving a mark.

If they occur in several locations of the body, they can also be present in different organs, creating potential danger for bleeding. Large hemangiomas can cause bleeding and anemia.

Hemangiomas can cause complications in the following circumstances:

- If they grow rapidly
- If they cause airway obstruction
- If they are bleeding
- If they are ulcerated and get infected
- If they obstruct vision, causing a lazy eye

Port-wine stain. These are dark-red or purple areas on the face, trunk, or extremities. They are permanent vascular birthmarks from birth. Large port-wine stains on the face, involving the eyelid, can be a sign of *Sturge-Weber syndrome*, which can be associated with seizures. Sturge-Weber syndrome is a rare neurological condition. It also can be associated with developmental delay.

Pigmented birthmarks. These birthmarks are present in different sizes, with pigment overgrowth.

The most common pigmented spots are called nevi. They are usually small and cause no trouble. But some birthmarks have the potential to become malignant, particularly large ones and those that are very dark. It is a good idea to show these spots to the doctor before your child starts puberty.

You want to take your child to see the doctor in the following circumstances:

- If the pigmented spot is dark or black
- If the birthmark is changing color
- If it is changing size
- If it has irregular borders
- If it bleeds or has an ulcer

In case of color change, increasing size, irregular borders, bleeding or ulceration there is an urgency to see the doctor. If any of these changes occur, there can be a suspicion of *melanoma* (skin cancer). Your child probable will see a skin doctor (dermatologist).

Mongolian spots. These are bluish black spots that are often present in larger areas. They are mostly seen on the buttocks, lower back, shoulders. They are harmless. They can be confused with bruises.

Café au lait spots. These birthmarks are small light-brown spots, like café au lait. They can be present anywhere on the skin, for example, the armpit (axilla).

They are only significant if three or more of them can be seen. In that case, they can be the symptom of an underlying medical condition, so-called *neurofibromatosis*. That disease can affect the nervous system. So if you see three or more of these kinds of spots, take your child to the doctor.

White spots and small white areas can also indicate an underlying medical problem, *tuberous sclerosis*. That disease can cause seizures. So if your child has those white spots, a checkup with the doctor is necessary.

Nevus sebaceous. That is a hairless yellow-orange small plaque (slightly raised area). It usually occurs on the scalp and face. It can be present at birth or in the first few years.

There is also *linear nevus sebaceous syndrome* (LNSS). In that case, a large linear sebaceous nevus is present. Seizures, eye abnormalities, intellectual disability are common, but it can affect any other organs. Diagnosis is made from the symptoms. The condition is not inherited. Treatment is symptomatic.

Tethered cord. Increased pigmentation, hemangioma, soft tumor (lipoma), tuft of hair, dermal pit over the lower spine can be a sign of an underlying medical problem, called tethered cord. That means that the spinal cord is restricted and cannot move in the spinal canal. The result is nerve damage and can create problems with walking when the spinal cord grows, unless it is surgically released.

So if you see anything mentioned above, over the lower spine, **urgently** see the doctor.

In case of tethered cord, a neurologist, then a pediatric neurosurgeon is involved in the child`s care.

Treatment is surgery.

Bites

Dog bites, rabies
Important questions:

- Do you know the dog that bit your child?
- Has the dog received all the necessary shots, especially rabies?
- Was the dog provoked?
- Was the dog behaving strangely?
- When was the last time your child had a tetanus shot (DTaP, Tdap, DT, or Td)?

The most serious consequence of a dog bite is rabies. In that case, the dog that bit the child is infected with the rabies virus. That disease is deadly, affecting mostly the nervous system. Therefore, if a dog bit your child, observation of the dog by a veterinarian is necessary. Every effort should be made to find and observe the dog. If it was a strange dog, you need to call the police.

Other sources of wildlife rabies are bats, racoons, skanks, foxes, coyotes, bobcats, and mongoose.

If you find a bat in your child's room, go to the emergency room, even if no bite or scratch is seen.

Rabies is now rare in the US.

The time from the dog bite till the development of rabies can be from days to years, but most often it is one to three months.

Symptoms: The initial symptoms are fever, vomiting, headache, malaise. Strange sensation (paresthesia), irritability, and drooling develop. The most characteristic symptom is the fear of drinking (hydrophobia). If the child tries to drink, aspiration occurs.

The child can have paralysis. Seizures are common, and coma develops.

Treatment: Clean the wound with soap and water. After that, the wound needs to be irrigated for at least ten minutes.

If there is bleeding, put pressure on the area.

If the child has not had a tetanus shot in the past five years (even if he is fully immunized), he needs to have one. Take your child to the emergency room for wound care and to see whether a tetanus, a rabies shot, and rabies immunoglobulin is necessary.

Insect bites. The most common insect bites are from fire ants, bees, wasps, hornets, and mosquitoes.

They can cause local reactions with a bump, redness, and itching, but also can cause allergic reactions that can be serious. Swelling of the eyelids, lips, hands, and feet can develop, as well as trouble breathing and shock.

In that case, the child has a cold sweat, the extremities are cold, and there is a change of consciousness. The heart rate is fast, and the breathing is also fast and hard. Bluish color of the nails, lips, and face can develop. (See allergies: allergic reaction and change in consciousness, fast breathing, cold sweat.)

If a bite gets infected, the area is red, hot, and swollen. If there is a sign of infection, see the doctor.

Treatment: You can use a cold washrag for the local reaction.

Bees leave a stinger at the bite. Try to remove it without squeezing the area.

If your child had an allergic reaction previously, give your child an epinephrine shot (EpiPen) if you have it. After that, you can give an antihistamine like Benadryl, Claritin, Zyrtec, Allegra if the consciousness is not altered and the child does not vomit.

Then go to the emergency room, or call 911.

If the child had an allergic reaction before, he or she needs to have EpiPen (epinephrine) ready all the time.

An antihistamine should be available as well.

Spider bites. Spider bites can cause local reaction and infection. If the bite seems to be infected, go to the doctor.

But there are two dangerous spiders, the black widow spider and the brown recluse spider.

The black widow spider bite causes sharp pain, and a little blood can be present at the bite.

Muscle cramps, stomach pain, and vomiting are the symptoms. Shock can develop.

Go to the emergency room or call 911.

The brown recluse spider bite produces increasingly severe pain, fever, rash, joint pain, change of consciousness.

There is a severe local reaction. Go to the emergency room or call 911.

Scorpion bites. Some scorpion bites only cause local swelling, redness, pain, while others cause vomiting, muscle pain, convulsions, and collapse.

If your child got a scorpion sting, keep him or her quiet, and go to the emergency room. However, if the symptoms are severe, like convulsion, call 911.

Snake bites. Snake bites can cause local reactions and severe systemic reactions.

The local reactions are burning, pain, and swelling.

Systemic reactions develop rapidly. Vomiting, bleeding, general weakness, and trouble breathing are the symptoms. Shock can develop (see change in consciousness, fast breathing and cold sweat).

The diagnosis can be made by the burning pain and the imprint of the fangs. One or two puncture wounds or scratches can be seen.

In case of a snake bite, keep the child quiet, and call 911. Wash the bite with soap and water. Try to describe the size, color, and shape of the snake because that helps the doctor to choose the right antivenin, also called antivenom.

Human bites. Human bites can cause bleeding. Pressure needs to be applied to stop it.

Human bites often get infected. The wound needs to be cleaned as described above, under dog bites. After that take your child to the emergency room.

Mosquito bites. Mosquito bites are common. They can cause only local reactions with itching or severe disease (see mosquito transmitted diseases).

Use insect repellents.

Jellyfish sting. Jellyfish sting causes local reactions with pain and irritated marks on the skin. However, some jellyfish stings can cause whole-body (systemic) illness with vomiting, muscle pain, stomachache, or even seizure or coma.

Treatment: You can put some vinegar or alcohol on the area of the sting. If there is a severe reaction, call 911.

Biting. Biting usually starts between one to three years of age. It is not uncommon that a toddler bites another child or even you.

The child can bite because he is teething, exploring by putting things in his mouth, or trying to get attention.

But it can happen also if the child is bored, unhappy, frustrated, upset, jealous, or wants something.

If your child bites, watch him closely, and try to prevent it. If he bit someone, say a firm no, show him your dissatisfaction, and maybe take a favorite toy away for a short while. Redirect him to another activity.

Praise him if there is no biting.

Some biting can occur during normal development, but this makes parents worried. If biting persists, it can be a sign of emotional and/or behavioral problem. See the doctor.

Biting at this early age does not imply the child's behavior in the future.

Bleeding problems

Children are active, often fall, and get bruises. But if they have too many bruises, or get bruises with no apparent reason, no history of fall or bumping to something, a bleeding problem can be suspected. The suspicion is stronger if the bleeding is heavy. A stronger-than-usual or longer-lasting bleeding after circumcision can be the first sign of a bleeding disorder. Other signs suspicious for a bleeding disorder can come from cuts, extracted teeth, nose bleed, heavy menstruation (metrorrhagia). Bleeding to the joints or muscles is a very significant symptom.

Important questions:

- Does the child get bruises easily without any cause?
- Does the child have significant bleeding after a minor injury or procedure?
- Does the bleeding last longer than expected?
- Does the bleeding recur frequently?
- Is there anybody in the family who has a similar problem or has a known bleeding disorder?

For proper blood clotting (coagulation), one needs, among other things, normal platelet count, Vitamin K, and certain clotting factors in the blood.

So some major causes of bleeding problems are low platelet count, Vitamin K deficiency, or inherited bleeding disorders.

The platelet count can be low from reaction to drugs and infections. However, the cause is often unknown, called *idiopathic thrombocytopenic purpura* (ITP).

Since some bleeding is due to *Vitamin K deficiency* and newborns have Vitamin K deficiency, it is very important that they receive a Vitamin K shot in the newborn nursery to prevent bleeding, including bleeding to the head (intracranial hemorrhage).

Vitamin K deficiency can develop from bowel and liver diseases. (See vitamins.)

In case of *inherited bleeding disorders*, certain blood clotting factors are low. The most important one is factor VIII, causing hemophilia. Since bleeding disorders are inherited, family history is very important.

There are two important inherited bleeding disorders: *hemophilia and von Willebrand disease.*

Symptoms: Excessive and prolonged bleeding from circumcision or tooth extraction that lasts much longer than expected. Easy bruising is characteristic.

A minor trauma can cause significant bleeding, even to the muscle or joint. Von Willebrand disease has a milder form as well. For all of these disorders, the diagnosis is made by laboratory tests.

Treatment:

ITP is treated with steroids.

In case of very low platelet count when there is a risk of severe bleeding, including bleeding to the brain (intracranial hemorrhage), platelet transfusion is needed. Vitamin K deficiency is treated with Vitamin K supplement.

The treatment of hemophilia and von Willebrand disease is the replacement of the clotting factors.

A specialist, hematologist, participates in the child's care.

Bladder infection (cystitis)

The symptoms, diagnosis, and treatment of bladder infections are the same as of urinary tract infections (UTI). (see urinary tract infection—UTI).

Blood pressure—high blood pressure (hypertension)

Blood pressure is usually measured when children have healthy checkups at three years of age.

High blood pressure in children is generally discovered during these exams.

High blood pressure can be a disease by itself, and then it is called primary hypertension. But high blood pressure in children is usually secondary to an underlying cause.

An elevated blood pressure measurement can be caused by anxiety about visiting the doctor, worrying about shots.

Therefore, repeated measurements are necessary to see if the child, in fact, has high blood pressure.

Common causes of high blood pressure:

- Kidney diseases are the most frequent causes of high blood pressure in children (congenital or acquired).
- Heart disease, like narrowing of the main artery in the body, called aorta (*coarctation of aorta*).
- Problem with the adrenal gland—excessive glucocorticoid hormone secretion (*Cushing's syndrome*) or with the thyroid gland—overproduction of the thyroid hormone (*hyperthyroidism*)
- There is a rare tumor called *pheochromocytoma* that causes high blood pressure by secreting certain hormones. Anxiety, a flushed face, sweating, headache, and fast heartbeats are the symptoms. Treatment is surgery.
- Obesity is a predisposition for high blood pressure.

Treatment of hypertension:

- Low-salt diet
- Low-calorie diet if the child is overweight
- Exercise

- Medication that lowers the blood pressure if it is necessary
- Treating the primary disease causing the high blood pressure, a cardiology consult might be necessary

Blood in the urine (hematuria)

Blood in the urine can be visible, but most of the time, it can only be detected with urine test and seen under a microscope (red blood cells).

Some causes of hematuria:

- Acute poststreptococcal glomerulonephritis (see below).
- Infections (see urinary tract infections).
- Hemolytic uremic syndrome (see diarrhea).
- Henoch-Schonlein purpura (see stomachache).
- Kidney stones (nephrolithiasis).
- Systemic lupus erythematosus (see joint pain with systemic disease).
- Trauma

Acute poststreptococcal glomerulonephritis

This condition develops approximately two weeks after an untreated or not properly treated streptococcal infection (see sore throat).

This kidney disease causes high blood pressure, blood, and protein in the urine.

If it is severe, it can cause kidney (renal) failure.

A blood test helps to make the diagnosis.

Treatment:

- Penicillin to eradicate the streptococcus
- Symptomatic treatments
- Control blood pressure with medication

Bluish discoloration—cyanosis

If the child's skin, lips, around the lips, and nail beds are dusky, that is called cyanosis. That means that the body does not get enough oxygen. The exception is if the color is caused by cold. Newborn babies are bluish right after birth. Their hands can be bluish later as well, if not kept warm.

Causes of cyanosis:

- Respiratory problems like upper airway obstruction from choking (see choking)
- Croup (see cough, respiratory problems, respiratory distress)
- Epiglottitis (see cough, respiratory problems, respiratory distress)
- Diphtheria (see infectious diseases of childhood)
- Lung diseases (see cough, respiratory problems, respiratory distress) like bronchitis, bronchiolitis, pneumonia, asthma, etc.
- Heart problems like congenital cyanotic heart disease (see heart problems)
- A blood disorder called methemoglobinemia (see methemoglobinemia)
- Extreme cold
- Breath-holding spell (see behavioral problems and habits)
- Panic attack if it is severe (see behavioral problems and habits)

If the child has cyanosis, urgent medical care is always necessary. But suddenly developing cyanosis is an emergency. Call 911. In certain situations when there is no breathing or heartbeats, cardiorespiratory resuscitation (CPR) should be initiated and 911 called.

Broken bones—fractures

If a child has healthy bones, fracture usually occurs only with a bad fall or other significant injury.

But sometimes, even when the fall does not seem to be too significant, it still can cause a fracture, particularly of the small bones, like metacarpals in the hands and metatarsals in the feet.

Signs of broken bone: Swelling, pain, and restricted movements because of the pain. Often there is bruising in the area. Babies and small children cry when the broken bone is touched or moved.

Treatment: Rest, splint, cast, avoidance of using the affected extremity. The splint or cast needs to extend over the joint above and below the fracture. If the fracture is at the lower extremity, crutches are needed.

In the treatment of fractures, orthopedic surgeons are usually involved.

Treatments by orthopedic surgeons: application of a splint, cast, reset the bone, or rarely, surgery can be necessary.

If the child has a splint or a cast and suddenly experiences an increase in pain, there is a concern that he or she has *acute compartment syndrome*. That means that the vessels, nerves, and muscles are under pressure from swelling and can be damaged.

The symptoms are severe cramping pain, and sometimes numbness. Acute compartment syndrome is an emergency.

Loosen the splint and go to the emergency room.

Treatment is surgery by an orthopedic surgeon to release the affected tissues from the pressure.

There is also a *chronic exertional compartment syndrome*.

This condition usually affects the lower leg secondary to exercise.

The symptoms are cramping pain, sometimes numbness during exercise.

The pain gets worse if the child continues the exercise.

Treatment is physical therapy and making changes in the physical activity. If there is no improvement and the symptoms are severe, the child might need to see an orthopedic surgeon. Surgery is a possibility.

Rib fracture. The child with rib fracture has sharp pain that is increasing with breathing. There is pain with compression of the chest bone (sternum) or rib cage as well.

Pneumothorax (ptx) can develop (see cough, respiratory problems, respiratory distress); therefore, a chest x-ray (CXR) is necessary.

Treatment is usually only pain management.

Collarbone (clavicle) fracture. Fracture of the clavicle is not uncommon, particularly during birth.

Symptoms are pain, swelling, and a bump when the fracture is healing.

Diagnosis: physical exam and x-ray.

Treatment: usually no treatment is necessary. If the fracture is painful, immobilization of the arm by pinning the sleeve to the cloth can be done.

Colles fracture. Colles fracture is the most common wrist fracture. It occurs most often when the child falls and lands on an outstretched hand.

Symptoms:

- Severe pain that gets worse when gripping or moving the hand or wrist
- Swelling
- Tenderness
- Bruising
- Deformity

If your child has these symptoms, go to the emergency room.

Treatment is splint or cast, but severe injuries may require surgery.

Contact sports increase the risk of fracture in the wrist.

Prevention: have your child wear wrist guards when playing high-risk sports.

Unexplained and frequent fractures need investigation. Often fractures bring up the possibility of child abuse.

Stress fracture. Stress fracture is a tiny crack in a bone. It is usually caused by repetitive strong movements, overuse. It most commonly affects the leg and the foot.
Symptoms: Initially slight pain that gets worse. If your child has pain when exercising, take him or her to the doctor.
Diagnosis is often made with MRI.
An orthopedic surgeon is generally consulted.
Treatment:

- Rest
- Ice
- Brace
- Crutches
- Surgery if necessary

Resume the sports activities slowly.

Bullying

Bullying is an act when a child repeatedly picks on another child.

Bullying can be physical, verbal, or social. Cyberbullying is another form of bullying.

Children who are bullied can have long-term effects. It can affect the child's school performance, it can make him depressed, and even suicide attempts occurred as a consequence of bullying.

Bullies often have problems in school or at home. They might be physically abused.

Both the child who is bullied and the bully need help. Parents need to talk to their child to find out what is going on.

If your child is bullied, ask him if there is any bullying going on in his class. Ask how children behave in his class and if he was ever bullied.

If he is bullied, reassure him that it is not his fault and that he has your full support. Encourage him to make friends and participate in activities he likes. Joining a sports team can be helpful.

Let school officials like his teacher and school counselor know about the problem, and work with them to solve it. Involve the parents of the bully.

If your child is the bully, ask him why is he bullying others and what is the reason for it. Teach him empathy, and tell him why bullying is wrong. Talk to school personnel as well.

Burns

Depending on the severity of the burn, first-, second- and third-degree burns are distinguished.

It is a first-degree burn if the affected area is only red. Most sunburn are first-degree burns.

In case of second-degree burn, there is redness and blisters.

Third-degree burn is the most severe, when grayish necrotic skin can be seen.

Important questions:

- How did the burn occur?
- How old is the child?
- How extensive is the burn?
- What body parts are burned?

The doctor evaluates the burn to see what degree burn the child has.

The child's age is important. The younger the child, the more severe the burn is.

The extent of the burn is calculated by the percentage of the affected total body surface.

Burn of the face, neck, groin area, hands, and feet are considered more serious. If the burn is severe, go to the emergency room, or call 911.

If the burn is not severe, place the burned area under clean cold running water promptly, and call the doctor.

Chemical burns need to be treated the same way.

The usual treatments are pain medications, plenty of fluids, and antiseptic cream.

Chemical burn of the eye is an emergency. Start irrigating the eye with plenty of water, and call 911.

Inhalation injury from direct heat or steam creates a dangerous situation, affecting the airways.

Call 911, because establishment of an airway with intubation is lifesaving.

Prevention of burns is extremely important.

Be sure that your child does not receive a burn from hot water, soup, coffee, tea, or your cigarette. Prevent him or her from touching the oven, iron, curling iron, or playing with the fireplace, matches, or fireworks. Cover the electric outlets, and keep matches in a safe place. Teach your child safety. To prevent sunburns, do not expose your baby to direct sun. Use sunscreens if sun exposure is expected. The sunscreen should contain at least PABA 30.

Canker sore (aphthous stomatitis)

If a child has canker sore, he has small, painful ulcers in his mouth. They are often seen inside of the lips and on the tongue. It usually resolves in one to two weeks.

Cat scratch disease

It is caused by a bacteria called *Bartonella henselae*.

If your child has a cat or plays with cats and develops symptoms like malaise, fatigue, headache, and develops lumps (enlarged lymph nodes), it is likely that he or she got the disease by a cat scratch or bite. Fever can develop, and the area of the scratch or bite can get infected. If your child has these symptoms, see the doctor. Less commonly, the disease can affect certain organs, including the eyes. Diagnosis is made by blood test.

Therapy is an antibiotic, azithromycin.

Change in consciousness, fast breathing, cold sweat—shock

Shock is a condition when the body does not get enough oxygen. It is a life-threatening end stage of different conditions.

The most common causes of shock are the following:

- Severe trauma, including spinal cord injury (neurologic)
- Severe blood or fluid loss (hypovolemic)
- Severe heart failure (cardiogenic)
- Severe infection (sepsis)
- Severe allergic reaction (anaphylactic)

The symptoms of shock are as follows:

Initially the child is anxious, then agitated, confused, very thirsty. The skin is pale, feet are cold, the heartbeat is fast. Nausea and vomiting can be present.

As the condition progresses, the child is less responsive and can lose consciousness.

The skin can be mottled or bluish. The child has a cold sweat. When the nail bed is pressed, the color does not return to normal in two seconds as it should (poor capillary refill). The breathing is fast, and the blood pressure is low.

In case of severe allergic reaction (anaphylactic shock), the child is also itching, has swelling of the eyelids, lips, hands, feet, or any other part of the body and may have an allergic rash. If insect bite is the cause, there is also swelling at the site of the bite.

Treatment: If there is suspicion of shock, call 911. Keep the child flat on her back, and turn the head to the side. Do not move him or her if there is any suspicion of head, neck, or spine injury.

IV fluid therapy and oxygen are the cornerstone of treatment. Much fluid is needed for the treatment of hypovolemic shock, much less for cardiac shock, so as not to overload the heart.

For the treatment of anaphylactic shock, epinephrine and steroids are also necessary.

Chest deformities

Pigeon chest (pectus carinatum). The chest bone (sternum) is protruding. Pigeon chest does not cause any problem.

Funnel chest (pectus excavatum). The chest bone has depression. It usually does not cause problems, unless the depression of the chest bone is extremely deep. In that case, the child can have difficulty breathing if a respiratory ailment, like asthma, is also present.

Horizontal depression of the rib cage. This depression in the front and at the side can be a sign of vitamin D deficiency (rickets).

Barrel-shaped chest. This can develop if the child has severe asthma for a long time.

Chest pain

It is not rare that a child complains of chest pain, but heart problems as the cause are rare.

Important questions:

- When did the pain start?
- Is the pain recurring? If the answer is yes, how often does the pain recur?
- Where is the pain located?
- Does it radiate anywhere?
- How bad is the pain?
- What kind of pain is it? Does it feel like pressure, squeezing and sticking?
- Did the child sweat?
- How long does the pain last?
- Is the pain related to breathing, coughing?
- Is the pain related to movements?
- Has the pain started or gotten worse with exercise?
- Does the child have a fever?
- Does the child have vomiting?
- Does the child feel a fast and hard heartbeat like his heart jumps out of his chest?
- Are there any other complaints?
- Did the child swallow a foreign body or take pills?
- Has the child had any injury?
- Is the child under stress, or is there stress in the family (death, serious illness, divorce)?
- Is there anybody in the family who has chest pain?

Causes of chest pain:

- Inflammation of the esophagus (esophagitis)
  Esophagitis is the inflammation of the tube (esophagus) that delivers food from the throat to the stomach.

Symptoms are cough, heartburn, chest pain (behind the breastbone when eating), pain when swallowing, difficulty swallowing (dysphagia), and the food can get stuck in the esophagus.

If your child has chest pain, feels that the food is lodged in the esophagus, has shortness of breath, call 911.

- Gastroesophageal reflux (stomach acids backing up into the esophagus)
- Allergy (eosinophilic esophagitis)
- Alkali poisoning (see poisoning)
- Infection
- Certain oral medications

    Treatment depends on the cause

- Foreign body in the esophagus. Symptoms are pain and trouble swallowing. That is an emergency. Go to the emergency room or call 911. (See foreign body.)
- Pneumonia, pleuritis. Symptoms are cough, often fever, and chest pain when the child takes a deep breath. Shortness of breath can develop. In that case, it is an emergency. Go to the emergency room or call 911. (See cough, respiratory problems, respiratory distress.)
- Pneumothorax (PTX)

    Pneumothorax is a condition in which some of the tiny pouches of the lung, filled with air (alveoli), burst, and air gets into the chest cavity. Symptoms are sharp chest pain and trouble breathing. Severe asthma is a predisposition for pneumothorax (see cough, respiratory problems, respiratory distress). Pneumothorax is a true emergency. Call 911.

- Asthma

    In case of asthma, the chest pain is located in the front. The cough is severe. Breathing can be difficult, in which case urgent medical care is necessary. (See cough, respiratory problems, respiratory distress.)

- Some heart conditions can cause chest pain. If the heart does not get a sufficient amount of oxygen (myocardial ischemia), like from narrowing of the coronary artery (angina), or obstruction (myocardial infarction). In these conditions, the pain is located in the middle of the chest and often radiates to the back, left shoulder, left arm. Exercise can provoke the development of pain. These conditions are rare in the pediatric age.

- Fast irregular heartbeats (arrhythmia) can cause chest pain, like supraventricular tachycardia (SVT). (See heart problems.)
- Infection, inflammation of the membrane around the heart also can cause chest pain (pericarditis). It can be caused by bacteria, viruses, but also diseases, like lupus and juvenile rheumatoid arthritis (see joint pain with systemic disease).
- Chest wall pain can be secondary to injury or muscle overuse.
- Costochondritis (inflammation at the rib cartilage) causes pain at the ribs.
- Viral infection can cause chest pain (pleurodynia). The child has severe chest pain at the lower chest, often only on one side. Movements can cause sharp pain. It usually lasts for one week, but relapses can occur. Treatment is anti-inflammatory drugs, like ibuprofen.
- Acute episodes of sickle cell disease can cause severe chest pain. It requires urgent medical attention. Go to the emergency room or call 911.
- Stress is a frequent cause of chest pain.

Treatment: Every child with chest pain needs to see the doctor. However, severe chest pain with difficulty breathing or color change is an emergency. Call 911.

The treatment of chest pain depends on the specific cause.

Child abuse and neglect

Child abuse is the mistreatment of a child.
The abuse can be physical, emotional and sexual.
Physical abuse is violence that harms the child.
Emotional abuse can be rejection or threat of violence.
Sexual abuse means sexual exploitation of a child.
Signs of physical abuse are bruises, burns, fractures.
Signs of emotional abuse are sleeping problems, change of behavior.

Signs of sexual abuse are genital injury, sexually transmitted disease, and when a child's sexual behavior is more mature than his or her age.

Neglect is failure to provide adequate food, cloth, shelter.

Signs of neglect are: FTT (failure to thrive), Inadequate clothing and medical care.

Child Protective Services deal with child abuse and neglect.

Choking

Prevention is most important.

Infants and toddlers should not eat alone. They should not eat or drink lying down. They should not walk or run with food in their mouth.

They should not get popcorn, nuts, hard candy, or gum. They should not eat a piece of apple, grape, cherry, carrots, celery, chunk of meat, or hot dogs because of the choking hazard.

Toys need to be checked to be sure that they do not have small pieces that can be taken out and they do not have batteries.

Children can choke from foreign bodies or from diseases, like croup, epiglottitis (see cough, respiratory problems, respiratory distress.), diphtheria (see infectious diseases of childhood). If the airway is fully obstructed, the child chokes. He or she cannot speak, cough, or get air. The face turns purple, and the child loses consciousness (see foreign bodies).

Treatment is dependent on the cause. The method of foreign body removal depends on the child's age.

Emergency removal of foreign bodies is taught with basic life support (CPR). If you are trained in CPR, start the treatment right away, and call 911.

Concussion

Children often fall and bump their heads. They play contact sports like football, soccer, baseball, basketball and get head injuries. Concussion is often the consequence.

Important questions:

- What happened?
- How did he get injured? What were the mechanics?
- Did he lose consciousness? If the answer is yes, how long was he out? Was he confused?
- Does he remember what happened? Was he oriented in space (places), time (events), and person (people)?
- Did he remember commonly known facts?
- Who was with him, and what did they say?
- Was he able to get up on his own?
- Was he able to walk? Was the walk normal or wobbly?
- Was he dizzy?
- Did he vomit?
- Did he have a headache?
- Was there any problem with his vision?
- Was his ear ringing?
- Has he had a concussion before?

Frequent symptoms are loss of consciousness, unsteady walk, drowsiness, dizziness, headache, vomiting. The child often does not remember what happened.

The most important thing is not to go back to the activity that caused the concussion too soon. The child needs to be checked by a doctor.

If the concussion is secondary to a serious injury, keep the child laying on the ground. Do not move him or her, be sure that the head does not move to prevent neck injury, and call 911.

After concussion, it is important that the child avoid physical and mental exercises as long as the doctor recommends it. Often the child sees a neurologist or a specialist of sports medicine. Follow-up care is very important because it needs to be seen that the symptoms are improving and whether help is needed to return to school. After concussion, initial reduction in physical and cognitive activity can be beneficial to recovery, but prolonged restrictions can have a negative effect. Students with concussion may need academic adjustments and modifications in school. Parents need to keep close contact with the school and the doctor.

Most students return to school within two to five days, but there are students who need more time. These are students who had more symptoms and more severe symptoms.

Students should be performing at their academic baseline before returning to sports. Return to play should be a gradual process. Start with a light activity, like light walking. If he has no symptoms, gradually increase the physical activity until he is ready to go back to play his sport.

Traumatic brain injury

Traumatic brain injury is damage of the brain from trauma. The important questions and the symptoms are the same as with concussion. MRI or CT scans are indicated. The child with TBI can have academic problems.

Constipation

Constipation is defined as lack of regular bowel movements. The child has fewer than three bowel movements a week, and the stools are very hard and hard to pass them. The stools get hard, and when the child goes to the toilet to have a bowel movement, it hurts. The hard stools can cause cuts (fissures) at the rectal area. The fissures can cause local bleeding. Also, because the fissure is painful, the child will withhold the stool. The constipation can be temporary and chronic.

Constipation can also cause hemorrhoids (see below).

Important questions:

- When was the last bowel movement?
- How often does the baby or child have bowel movements?
- What do the stools look like, and what is their consistency?
- Is there any blood in the stool?
- Is there any rectal fissure?
- Have your child symptoms been occasional or continuous? Are there any soiling of his underwear?
- Was there any problem with toilet training?
- Is there a family history of constipation?
- If a baby is constipated, is he or she nursing or taking formula?
- How old was the child when the constipation started?
- Is the urination okay?

Breastfed babies sometimes do not have stools for three to four days. If the baby is otherwise okay, that is normal.

Formula-fed babies usually have bowel movement every day or every other day. But two to three bowel movements a day are also normal.

Parents often complain that the baby has constipation when he or she strains when having bowel movements. Straining is common and does not mean constipation if the stools are regular.

Some foods make the stool harder, like carrots, rice, apples, and bananas.

If constipation is a problem, decrease or temporarily stop these foods.

Other foods can make the stools softer, like barley cereal, green vegetables, and fruits (with the exception of apples and bananas). Spinach is particularly helpful. You can give peaches to your baby.

Peaches, pears, strawberries, oranges, grapes, and melons can be given to children for constipation, but prunes help the most. Also, juices like orange, grape, tomato, and prune are useful.

You can make diet changes, but also call the doctor to ask the specifics.

Problem with toilet training is an important cause of constipation. If it starts too early, it is too harsh, and if the parents scold or punish the child for accidents, constipation can develop.

Some children fight toilet training. Be patient and wait. Stop the toilet training for a few weeks, and gently start again. Do not talk about frustration or inconvenience.

Hemorrhoid

Constipation can cause hemorrhoids. Hemorrhoids are swollen veins at the anus.

Symptoms are rectal pain, itching, and bleeding.

Treatment: Treat the constipation.

Talk to the doctor.

There are some serious medical conditions that can cause constipation, like meconium ileus and Hirschsprung disease (see below).

Meconium ileus

The first stools a newborn has are called meconium. They are thick and dark green.

In case of meconium ileus, the newborn has bowel obstruction secondary to a very thick meconium that he or she cannot expel.

Meconium ileus can be a sign of cystic fibrosis (see cough, respiratory problems, respiratory distress).

Symptoms are no passage of meconium, vomiting, and swollen belly (abdominal distention).

X-ray helps to make the diagnosis.

Treatment: The baby needs to be seen by a surgeon. The surgeon may try to solve the blockage with enema. If that does not help, the baby needs surgery.

Hirschsprung disease

In this disease, nerve cells are missing in the lower intestine. The result is constipation. The newborn may not be able to pass the meconium. Depending on the severity of the disease, it can cause bowel obstruction or enlargement of the colon (megacolon). Megacolon can cause inflammation of the bowel (enterocolitis), resulting in diarrhea, dehydration, and malnutrition. In a mild case, the only symptom is constipation. History reveals that the child has been having constipation since birth. The other important finding is that there is no stool in the rectum when the doctor does a rectal examination. With regular constipation, there is stool in the rectum, unless the child had a bowel movement right before the exam.

If your child has constipation, vomiting, and a swollen belly, go to the emergency room, or call 911.

Chronic constipation can cause urinary tract infections. If stool fills up the rectum, it can pressure the bladder, and the bladder cannot empty completely. The urine that stays in the bladder is a good media for bacteria to grow and cause infection.

Constipation also can lead to soiling of the clothing.

Soiling of the clothing (encopresis)

Encopresis means the passage of stool in an inappropriate place (most often clothing) after the age of toilet training, usually after four years of age.

Soiling of the clothing is often caused by constipation. The child does not have regular bowel movements, and the rectum gets full. Some of the feces spill over. Painful cracks at the rectum increase the accumulation of stools because of the pain when the child is trying to pass them. Soiling of the pants and wetting the pants can go together and can indicate emotional problems. In that case, a consultation with a psychologist is warranted.

Treatment of constipation

First, try to solve the constipation with diet change (see above). If that did not help, maybe a stool softener or laxative is needed. But before using a laxative, talk to the doctor. Sometimes a suppository or an enema is necessary. Do not use enema if your child has stomachache, vomiting, or swollen belly. It is good practice to have your child sit on the toilet every day at the same time. It helps to develop a habit to have regular bowel movements.

It is important to see the doctor to be sure that no underlying medical condition exists. Such a visit will also help you to manage the constipation and refer your child to a gastroenterologist if necessary.

In case of soiling of the clothing, you want to reassure your child of your support and the fact that the problem will go away. You need to explain that the maturation of the body is gradual. For some children, it happens sooner, and for others later. Therefore, the control of bowel movement differs from child to child. The child's cooperation is very important. When the clothing is soiled, do not show frustration or talk about inconvenience. You want to praise your child for any improvement.

Cough, respiratory problems, respiratory distress

Cough is a common symptom of many diseases.

It often represents "only a cold" or upper respiratory infection (URI) caused by different viruses, but can be caused by more severe diseases as well.

Important questions:

- How long has the child been coughing?
- Has the child been having a runny nose or nasal congestion?
- Has the child been having a fever? If the answer is yes, how high was the fever, and how was the temperature taken? What kind of thermometer was used?
- Has the cough been dry or productive? (Productive, congested cough means that the child coughs up phlegm.) If the child has a wet cough, maybe coughs up phlegm, what is the color? Is there any blood in the sputum?
- Does the cough sound like a dog barking?
- How frequent is the cough? How many coughs are there in a row?
- Has the child been having coughing spells?
- What part of the day is the cough the worst? Is it at night, in the early morning, or during the day?
- Has the child been waking up at night because of the cough?
- Is there any vomiting secondary to the cough?
- Has he or she had this kind of cough before? If the answer is yes, how many times, and how often has it recurred? How long did the cough last?
- Is the breathing okay? Is there any noise with the breathing? Is there any wheezing? Is the breathing normal or fast? Is breathing easy or hard? If the breathing is difficult, the child has retractions. In that case, there is pulling in under the neck, under the chest, or between the ribs. The more difficult the breathing is, the deeper the retractions are.

- Is there anybody around the child who has a similar cough?

Cough can be acute, lasting one to three weeks, or chronic, lasting longer than three weeks. The cough can be dry, barking, and wet. Children also can have coughing spells.

Children often are not able to cough up phlegm, but a productive cough sounds wet.

Acute cough is present in the following illnesses:

Common cold or upper respiratory infection (URI). This can cause cough, runny nose, and nasal congestion. Also influenza and many other viruses can cause these symptoms. Some infectious diseases like measles or rubella, also caused by viruses, display the symptoms of cough and runny nose.

Often fever, sore throat, pink eye, headache can be present as well.

Allergies can cause runny nose or nasal congestion and cough as well.

Barking cough. It is a very deep, hoarse cough, sounding like a dog's bark.

Barking cough is the characteristic symptom of croup, epiglottitis, tracheitis (see below).

All of these diseases can cause airway obstruction; therefore, a barking cough should always be taken seriously.

If the only symptom is the barking cough, the child needs to see the doctor.

But if there is any sign of respiratory problems, like noisy breathing, stridor (hoarse sound when the child is breathing in), he or she needs to go to the emergency room. However, if the stridor is heard all the time, there is pulling in (retraction) under the neck, the child is gasping for air, or any color change developed, call 911.

Croup. Croup is usually a viral disease. It can occur from infancy to five years of age.

Croup has the tendency to recur. It causes narrowing of the upper airways, which can be mild, moderate, or severe. Croup usually starts suddenly, often in the early morning.

The first sign is a dry, barking cough. Fever can be present.

The barking cough and often a rough noise with inspiration (stridor) are characteristic of croup.

If the croup is mild, the child may only have a barking (croupy) cough. If the illness is worse, the stridor can be heard. But when the croup is severe, the child has noisy and troubled breathing. There is pulling in under the neck and often below the rib cage. When the child gets anxious and cries, the breathing gets louder and harder. Try to keep the child calm. Give him plenty of fluids. Use a humidifier with cool mist, or run the hot water in the bathroom. Stay with your child. Do not put the humidifier close to your baby because it can make him cold.

Treatment is cool mist and usually steroid.

Every child with a croup needs to be checked by a doctor. However, if the breathing is impaired, go to the emergency room, or call 911.

Epiglottitis. Epiglottitis is similar to croup, but it is caused by bacterial infection. *Haemophilus influenzae* is the bacteria.

It is transmitted from person to person.

Epiglottitis is the infection and inflammation of the epiglottis.

Since the epiglottis is located above the voice box (larynx), preventing food getting to the airways, when it is swollen, the airway is compromised.

The child looks very sick, with high fever. He or she is sitting up to help the breathing, drooling, noisy, and heavy breathing are also present.

This disease is a true emergency. Call 911.

Treatment:

- Artificial airway (intubation), in which a tube is placed to the windpipe (trachea).

- Oxygen
- Intravenous (IV) (into the vein) antibiotic

Laryngitis. Laryngitis is a viral infection affecting the voice box (larynx).

Cough and hoarseness are the characteristic symptoms. Fever is also often present.

The treatment is symptomatic. Tylenol or ibuprofen can be given for the fever. The child needs to drink plenty of fluids and inhale cool mist (humidifier).

Tracheitis. Tracheitis is often a bacterial infection. The cause is most often a bacteria, called *Staphylococcus aureus.*

Tracheitis often starts as a viral illness, then high fever and respiratory distress develop, signaling the presence of a bacterial infection.

Symptoms are similar to croup, like barking cough and noisy breathing. The child also has a thick green sputum.

Go to the emergency room, or if the breathing is hard, call 911.

In case of tracheitis, the usual treatment for croup does not work.

Treatment is antibiotic, oxygen, and often artificial airway (intubation), when a tube is placed to the windpipe (trachea).

Coughing spells and vomiting. If a child has a cough that is getting worse and worse, culminating in a burst of cough, coughing spell, or if he or she has trouble getting air because of the continuous cough, whooping cough is likely. The coughing spell often ends with a noise when the child inhales, called whoop. The whoop is not always present. Babies, for example, do not have the whoop, but they can stop breathing. Vomiting is also frequent after the coughing spell, making the whooping cough diagnosis more likely (see infectious diseases of childhood).

Other diseases can also cause coughing spells and vomiting, like bronchiolitis, reactive airway disease (RAD), and asthma.

If the cough is very bad, it can cause the child to develop some small red dots on the face or eyes. Those are blood spots called petechiae. They do not change color when pressed and go away with time.

Bronchiolitis. Bronchiolitis is a disease of the small tubes (bronchioles) in the lung.

It is usually caused by viruses. *Respiratory syncytial virus* (RSV) is the most common virus causing bronchiolitis. It usually occurs from fall to spring.

Human metapneumovirus is another virus causing bronchiolitis, usually in the winter and spring. It also can cause bronchitis and pneumonia.

Symptoms can be similar to the symptoms of asthma., coughing, coughing spells, wheezing, difficulty breathing. Fever, nasal congestion, and vomiting are also common. Bronchiolitis can cause severe respiratory distress.

Treatment of bronchiolitis:

Plenty of fluids (babies need Pedialyte or similar liquids since regular water can be harmful in larger amounts at this age) and cool-mist humidifier. Do not place the humidifier close to the baby because it can make him or her cold.

If your child has coughing spells or wheezing, see the doctor. If your child has difficulty breathing, go to the emergency room, or call 911.

Bronchitis. Bronchitis is the infection of the larger tubes in the lung (bronchi). Bronchitis is most often caused by viruses, but bacteria can cause it too. Often there is sputum production.

Treatment depends on the cause.

Pneumonia. If the child has high fever or the fever does not break, only temporarily with fever reducers, and there is a significant cough, pneumonia is suspected. However, one can have pneumonia without fever, called walking pneumonia, usually caused by viruses.

Pneumonia is the infection and inflammation of the lung.

It can be caused by viruses, bacteria, and, less commonly, by other agents.

It can develop gradually from another infection, like a cold, bronchitis, or bronchiolitis, or it can start abruptly.

Symptoms are fever, cough, fatigue. Fast and hard breathing can develop.

The diagnosis is made by history and physical exam, but sometimes a chest x-ray is necessary.

Treatment: plenty of fluids, fever reducers, but in case of bacterial pneumonia, antibiotic therapy is necessary as well.

Recurrent pneumonia can indicate an aspirated foreign body or low immunity (immunodeficiency). Foreign body aspiration happens when the child swallows wrong and food gets to the windpipe (trachea then to the bronchi). Also, small objects can get there (see foreign bodies). Cystic fibrosis also can cause recurrent pneumonia. If the membrane around the lung (pleura) gets infected too (*pleuritis*), the child will have chest pain when breathing in.

Pleural effusion. Pleural effusion is a complication of pneumonia.

Fluid accumulates in the so-called pleural cavity. The pleural cavity is the potential space between the two layers of the thin membrane called pleura. The outer layer of the pleura is attached to the inside of the chest wall. The inner layer covers the lungs.

Viruses, bacteria, and sometimes other agents can cause pleural effusion.

Tuberculosis can cause pleural effusion as well.

If fluid accumulates in the pleural space (pleural effusion), the child can be sick for a long time, weeks to months.

The symptoms are fever that can last for a longer time, cough, and often troubled breathing.

The diagnosis is made by history, physical exam, chest x-ray, and the analysis of the pleural fluid, obtained by needle stick and aspiration from the pleural space.

Aggressive antibiotic therapy, sometimes surgery, and video-assisted thoracoscopic surgery (VATS) is necessary.

A chronic cough is present in the following diseases:

Asthma. Asthma is a chronic lung disease causing cough and often a characteristic noisy breathing, called wheezing.

The airways get narrow and swollen inside. There is inflammation in the lung and the production of thick white mucus. If these changes are more severe, the child develops an *asthma attack* with shortness of breath. It is hard for the child to exhale. The more severe the attack is, the more troubled the breathing is. But it is important to know that one can have an asthmatic attack without wheezing. In that case, only the heavy breathing is present. That condition can be even more severe than the one with wheezing.

Asthma symptoms often recur and also can last for a long time.

A child who has asthma usually coughs at night and during exercise.

An asthma attack is often triggered by allergens (substances that the child is allergic to), infections, viral or bacterial, cold air, exercise, and emotional upsets.

Frequent allergens are house dust, insects, molds, animal dander, pollens, and foods.

Foods most commonly causing allergies are nuts, eggs, cow's milk, shellfish, fish, wheat, soy.

Important questions:

- How long has the child been coughing?
- Has he had any wheezing?
- How long has he or she had asthma?
- Does he or she have coughing spells?
- Does he or she have a cough at night?
- Does he or she have a cough while exercising?
- Does the child have sputum? If the answer is yes, is it white?

- Is there any problem with breathing? If the answer is yes, how often, and how bad is it?
- If the child has asthma, how many nights does he or she wake up coughing in a week?
- How many times a week does he or she have trouble breathing?
- How many days of school are missed because of asthma?
- Does he or she have a nebulizer or an inhaler? If an inhaler is used, is it attached to an AeroChamber?
- How often does he or she have to use an inhaler or nebulizer?
- If an inhaler is used, how long did it last before he or she bought a new one?
- Does he or she have enough asthma medication?
- Has he or she ever been hospitalized with asthma?
- Has he or she ever been in an intensive care unit (ICU) with asthma? If the answer is yes, was he or she ever intubated?
- Is there anybody in the family with asthma?

Again, the symptoms of asthma are chronic cough, often wheezing, and nasal congestion from nasal allergy (allergic rhinitis), and shortness of breath in case of asthma attack.

An acute severe asthma attack that does not respond to initial therapy is called *status asthmaticus*.

The diagnosis of asthma is made from the history and physical examination, but pulmonary function tests are also helpful. Those tests determine how well the lungs work. The most common test is spirometry. The child blows into a tube connected to a machine called spirometer (see tests, procedures, surgeries).

A peak flow meter can help to evaluate the present status of asthma. The child needs to blow into a tube as hard as he or she can. This device measures how much air moves out of the lung with one strong exhalation. If it is decreasing, that shows that the asthma is worsening, or maybe an attack is coming,

Some children will grow out of asthma.

Therapy:

The child needs to drink plenty of fluids to decrease the thickness of the sputum.

Medications are bronchodilators like epinephrine, albuterol, Xopenex. These kinds of medications open up the little tubes (bronchioles) in the lung. These medications are often delivered by nebulizers or inhalers.

A nebulizer is a machine that delivers medications in a form of aerosol. Albuterol is commonly used.

An inhaler is a small device delivering puffs from the medication. Often a so-called AeroChamber is used. That is like a tube and is attached to the inhaler. The role of the AeroChamber is to channel the medicine more efficiently into the airways.

If the cause is allergy, that needs to be treated with antihistamine like Claritin, Zyrtec, Allegra, etc. Often an allergist is involved in the child's care.

If the child has an asthma attack, steroid treatment is often necessary.

If the cause is a bacterial infection, an antibiotic is used.

For long-term treatment of asthma, often a steroid inhaler is used like Flovent, Pulmicort, and Qvar, and it can be combined with a long-acting bronchodilator as well. Advair and Symbicort are such combinations.

Allergic rhinitis is treated with saline nasal spray and steroid nasal spray. Antihistamines are also often used.

A child with asthma needs regular follow-ups. If the symptoms of asthma are getting worse or not controlled, the child needs to see the doctor. A child with an asthma attack needs immediate medical attention, so he or she needs to see the doctor urgently. If the attack is severe, go to the emergency room, or call 911.

A pulmonologist is often involved in a child's care who has severe asthma.

Reactive airway disease (RAD). The symptoms and treatment of reactive airway disease are pretty much like asthma. Actually, until the diagnosis of asthma is made, the condition is often called reactive airway disease.

Cystic fibrosis (CF). Cystic fibrosis is a serious chronic disease.

In CF, thick mucus is produced that can harm the lungs, pancreas, sometimes the liver.

The salt level of the sweat is high.

Since the lungs cannot get rid of the mucus, respiratory infections like bronchitis, bronchiolitis, and pneumonia are frequent, often causing respiratory distress.

Another complication is dehydration secondary to salt and fluid loss.

The child often has a cough, and it can be persistent.

The stools are greasy and foul-smelling. Since some enzymes made by the pancreas are lacking, the fat absorption is impaired. Consequently, there will be some vitamin deficiency. The level of fat-soluble vitamins such as Vitamin A, D, E, and K are low.

The impaired absorption of food from the bowels leads to inadequate nutrition; therefore, the child's weight lags behind.

The diagnosis is made by a laboratory test, measuring the chloride content of the sweat. If the child has cystic fibrosis, the level is high.

The disease is inherited.

Lately, the newborn screening test includes cystic fibrosis.

Treatment:

- No specific treatment is available.
- Antibiotic treatment is used to fight bacterial infection.
- Some medications are used to make the mucus thinner.
- Chest physiotherapy can help to bring up the mucus.
- Pancreatic enzymes are given to improve digestion.
- Increased amounts of fluids are given, and vitamins.

To prevent infections, pneumonia shots are given, and yearly influenza shots.

Bronchiectasis. Bronchiectasis is the dilatation of one or more tubes (bronchi) in the lung. Infection is often present.

Symptoms are chronic cough and sputum. The child can have fever, and that can recur.

The diagnosis is made by chest x-ray.

Treatment is antibiotics, but surgery can be necessary too.

Tuberculosis (TB). Tuberculosis is a contagious chronic disease.

It is caused by a bacteria, called *Mycobacterium tuberculosis.*

The incubation period is one to six months (from the time of the infection until the appearance of symptoms).

Tuberculosis most often affects the lungs, but any other part of the body can be involved.

The disease spreads by droplets from the sputum of an infected person.

The infection can be latent, without symptoms. It can spread locally or by the bloodstream.

Important questions:

- Is there anybody in the family who ever had TB?
- Has the child been in contact with anybody who has TB?
- Was the child born in a country where TB is common?
- Has he or she spent more than two weeks in a country where TB is common?
- Has the child been in contact with someone who spent a longer time in a country where TB is common?
- Has the child been in contact with anybody who spent time in jail, is addicted to drugs, or has HIV?

The symptoms of lung infection are chronic cough, coughing up blood, night sweat, fatigue, elevated temperature, weight loss.

Often the first manifestation of TB is pneumonia, which does not respond to the usual antibiotics.

If tuberculosis is present for a long time, cavities can develop in the lung.

Lymph nodes also can be enlarged.

Meningitis can develop as well (see vomiting).

The diagnosis is made by history (which is very important), physical exam, chest x-ray, and specific tests for tuberculosis. These tests are the tuberculin test and the QuantiFERON Gold.

Tuberculin contains TB antigens that are injected into the skin of the child's forearm. It is checked forty-eight to seventy-two hours later. If the site of the injection gets red and raised, that is suggestive of TB. If a child received BCG shot, the tuberculin test also can be positive (red and raised area), like he or she would have TB. (See below.) If the tuberculin test is negative, that means that the child probably does not have TB.

Lately, there is a blood test QuantiFERON Gold (Interferon Gamma Release Assay, or IGRA), which helps to distinguish whether TB or BCG shot caused the positive TB test (red and raised area of the skin). If the IGRA test is positive, that means that TB is likely. If the test is negative, that means that the child has no infection.

The TB tests will turn positive two to ten weeks after infection.

The diagnosis is confirmed if the germ that is causing TB is found in the sputum.

Treatment: Antitubercular drug therapy. The treatment usually includes multiple drugs and can last for years. Even if there is only suspicion that the child has TB, at least six months of therapy is necessary.

The vaccine to prevent TB, called BCG. It has been used in many countries, but not in the USA. There is one disadvantage in using the vaccine. As mentioned above, the tuberculin test that is negative when a healthy child is tested turns positive after the BCG shot is given, as if the child had TB.

Another germ, *Mycoplasma Bovis*, also can cause tuberculosis but much less frequently.

The infection gets transmitted to the child from infected cattle by unpasteurized milk or dairy products.

Children and their parents can get infected in countries where cattle are infected.

In children, the lymph nodes get infected and enlarged on the neck, the bowels get infected, but it can cause infection in other locations as well.

Meningitis can develop too.

Gastroesophageal reflux disease (GERD). GERD can cause chronic cough (see vomiting).

Children with low immunity (immunodeficiency) can develop diseases that can cause chronic cough (see sickness all the time—immunodeficiency).

Cuts and lacerations

You need to stop the bleeding by keeping pressure on the area, preferably with a piece of gauze or clean cloth. When the bleeding stops, clean the wound with soap and water. Do it gently to avoid the recurrence of the bleeding. Cover the cut with a bandage to keep it clean, but first use some antibiotic ointment like Neosporin so the bandage does not stick in the wound.

For deeper cuts, you need to seek medical attention within six hours in case stitches are needed. After six hours, stitches only can be placed after some tissues are removed, often by a surgeon.

Your child needs medical attention in the following circumstances:

- If the cut is deep, or you are not sure about it.
- If there is foreign body in the wound.
- If the wound is dirty.
- If the bleeding does not stop after ten minutes of firm pressure, or the blood soaks through the bandage. However, if the bleeding is heavy, call 911.
- If there is a red streak from the wound.
- If your child has a fever.
- If the pain is getting worse.
- If there is redness and swelling in the area.
- If your child has not had tetanus shot, DTaP, DT, Tdap, or Td in the past five years.

For bone, joint, and tendon injuries, an orthopedic surgeon is involved in the treatment of the child.

It is very important to be sure that your child is protected against tetanus.

Tetanus. Tetanus or lockjaw is a life-threatening bacterial infection.

The germ called *Clostridium tetani* is very common in the soil. The soil gets contaminated by animal faces.

When wounds, particularly deep puncture wounds, and burns get contaminated, the bacterium produces a toxin, and the disease develops.

Incubation period is three to twenty-one days.

The hallmark of the symptoms is generalized painful muscle spasm.

Stiff neck and lockjaw develop and swallowing problem with consequent dehydration.

Breathing difficulty is common, and in severe cases, spine fracture can occur. Sweating, fast breathing (tachypnea), and irregular heartbeats (arrhythmia) are often present as well.

Newborns can get tetanus through the navel cord. Therefore, women after delivery should not get flowers or plants with soil because it can harm both the newborn and the mother.

Treatment is tetanus immune globulin, sedatives, and muscle relaxants.

Prevention is most important.

Active immunization is the most effective preventative measure. The immunization schedule includes tetanus shots in the form of DTaP, and Tdap. DT and Td also include tetanus shots.

It is very important to get all the shots and booster shots according to the schedule, and after that, to get a booster shot every ten years. However, if there is an injury, and the last tetanus shot was given five years before, the shot needs to be repeated. So it is important to know your child's immunization status.

After injury, a thorough wound cleaning is also important.

Bite wounds are a high risk of infection. They should be irrigated with plenty of water, left open to drain, and inspected daily for infection. If the laceration is caused by a dog bite, it is important to clean the wound with soap and water. After that, the wound needs to be irrigated with running water for at least ten minutes.

(See dog bites.) You need to get information about the dog, and take the child to the emergency room for wound care and to see whether a tetanus, a rabies shot, or rabies immunoglobulin is necessary. If it is an unknown dog, call the police.

If there is significant bleeding that does not stop, call 911.

Cystitis-bladder infection (see urinary tract infection-UTI)

Diaper rash, yeast diaper rash (monilia)

Diaper rash is usually caused by irritation from urine or stool.

Frequent diaper change can often prevent the development of diaper rash.

Also, applying a protective diaper rash cream after each diaper change is very useful.

A baby can also be sensitive to a certain diaper.

If you use a cloth diaper, be sure to rinse it thoroughly so no detergent stays on the diaper because that irritates the baby's skin (contact dermatitis).

Atopic dermatitis and eczema often show up as diaper rash.

Chubby babies often have red and peeling skin in the creases of the neck, armpits, and thighs (*intertrigo*). Frequent cleaning and removal of the sweat and other irritants help. Place a piece of gauze into the crease, and change it often.

Diaper rash often improves if exposed to air. Be sure that the temperature of the room is comfortable for the baby.

If you do all of these things and the diaper rash is not getting better, yeast infection can be the cause (*monilial diaper rash*).

If that is the case, beside the redness of a diaper rash, small bumps are also visible.

This kind of diaper rash is not uncommon in babies and is often accompanied by white spots on the tongue and inside the mouth (*thrush*). Contact your baby's doctor if the diaper rash is getting worse or not getting better after a few days. Also call if it looks bad, blisters or open sores are present, swelling is seen, or yeast infection is suspected. You want to call as well if you see white spots, white areas inside your baby's mouth, and it is always there, so it is not milk. The milk would come off. The treatment of yeast dermatitis is anti-yeast cream. The thrush is treated with anti-yeast liquid like nystatin.

Another type of diaper rash is located around the butthole (anus) called *perianal dermatitis*. The area is very red with a well-defined border. Itching, discomfort, and maybe a foul smell is present. The child often withholds the stool because of the pain.

The cause is a bacterial infection (*Streptococcus pyogenes* or *Staphylococcus aureus*).

If you see this kind of diaper rash, see the doctor soon.

Treatment is antibiotic.

Do not let your child bathe with anybody.

If the diaper rash is persistent and consists of red plaques with some scaling, a chronic inflammatory condition called *psoriasis* can be the cause.

Diarrhea

Parents sometimes complain that the baby has diarrhea, when in fact he or she does not. If there is only one or two stools a day, even if it is loose, that is not diarrhea. The number of bowel movements, the consistency, the color, the smell, and the presence of mucus or blood determines if a baby or child has diarrhea.

We can say that a baby has too many stools if there are more than eight a day on breastfeeding, more than three to four a day on formula feeding, and more than three per day for a child.

Breastfed babies often have watery stools. They often have four-six stools a day. If the color is yellow, there is no foul smell and no mucus or blood in the stool, it is normal.

Important questions:

- When did the diarrhea start?
- How many stools did the baby or child have? (If a baby has two small stools within fifteen minutes, that counts only as one.)
- What did the stools look like?
- What is the color?
- Are the stools foul-smelling?
- Have the stools had any mucus or blood?
- Is the stool shiny?
- Has the child had any vomiting?
- Has the child had any fever?
- Has the child had a stomachache?
- Is there anybody around the child who had diarrhea?
- Has the child traveled outside the USA lately? If the answer is yes, what country or countries he or she visited, and for how long?
- How many times did the child urinate during the past twenty-four hours, and when was the last time (see dehydration)?

Diarrhea and fever

If a child has diarrhea and fever, infection is likely. It can be caused by viruses, bacteria, parasites, and, rarely, fungal infections. Vomiting is common.

Viruses

Rotavirus. This is the most common virus causing diarrhea. It is more common in the winter months.

Incubation period is one to three days. The virus spreads from person to person through hand to mouth contact and contaminated objects.

Symptoms are fever, vomiting, watery diarrhea.

Treatment is clear liquids and BRAT diet (see below).

Immunization is available to prevent *Rotavirus* infection. Since the vaccine is given by mouth, and the virus is excreted in the feces and spreads to others (herd immunity), the number of infections has declined in general.

Norovirus. This is another major cause of diarrhea. It also can cause outbreaks. The origin is contaminated food or water, and it spreads from person to person.

Incubation period is twelve to forty-eight hours.

Symptoms are vomiting, watery diarrhea, abdominal cramps.

Treatment is clear liquids and BRAT diet (see below).

Bacteria

The bacteria most often causing diarrhea are *Shigella, Salmonella, E.coli, Campylobacter.*

Shigella dysentery. Shigella infection is most often spread from person to person, but the infection can be transferred by ingestion of contaminated food and water as well.

The incubation period varies from one to seven days.

Symptoms are bloody diarrhea, abdominal cramps, vomiting, and high fever. Babies and young children can get seizures from high fever.

Diagnosis is made by culturing the bacteria from the stool.

Treatment is antibiotics, but older children usually do not need therapy since the disease is self- limiting.

Salmonella infections. Chickens, ducks, reptiles, pet turtles can spread the disease. Incubation period is twelve to thirty-six hours.

Symptoms are fever, vomiting, abdominal pain, and watery or bloody diarrhea with mucus.

Diagnosis is made by culturing the bacteria from the stool.

Complications can develop, like pneumonia and bone infection (osteomyelitis).

The most serious form of salmonella infection is *typhoid fever*. It is transported from person to person. Incubation period is seven to fourteen days.

Besides the symptoms mentioned above, a rash can develop, and the disease can end with coma.

The disease can recur even after treatment. Treatment is antibiotics.

There are two vaccines to prevent typhoid fever. One is an inactive vaccine, a shot, which can be given to children two years and older. The other one is a live vaccine, capsules, and can be given to children who are six years and older. These capsules must be stored in a refrigerator but not in the freezer.

These vaccines are usually given before someone goes to a place where typhoid fever is common (East and Southeast Asia, the Caribbean, and Central and South America).

For other salmonella infections, antibiotics are usually not indicated, but for selected cases (infants and children who have problems with their immune system or have a severe infection).

There is another disease with similar name as typhoid fever, called typhus. This disease is caused by a different bacteria called *Rickettsia* (see typhus).

E. coli infection. Transmission of E. coli is from contaminated food, water, or sick persons. Incubation period is from ten hours to six days.

The child has loose, green, foul-smelling stools. Diagnosis is made by culturing the bacteria from stool.

Treatment: fluids and antibiotics in certain cases.

E. coli also can cause a more severe disease with bloody diarrhea. Rarely, it can also cause a disease called *hemolytic uremic syndrome* (*HUS*). This disease can cause anemia, low platelet count, and kidney failure. Therefore, if your child has bloody diarrhea, particularly with dark urine, decreased urine output, and/or if bruises are present, call the doctor right away, or go to the emergency room.

Travelers' diarrhea. Travelers' diarrhea is often caused by E. coli infection.

Symptoms are loose, watery stools, vomiting, stomachache, and fever. It can cause dehydration with symptoms of weakness, sunken eyes, dry coated tongue, and acetone smell in the breath (see dehydration).

Treatment:

- Rehydration (You can buy oral rehydration salt packages from the pharmacy before traveling. You can add that to water when needed.)
- Antibiotic when necessary

Prevention:

- Drink only bottled or boiled water. Use only bottled beverage.
- Practice good handwashing.

- Avoid ice and raw foods like salads.
- Eat fruits that have thick peel like bananas.
- If your child's diarrhea is severe, see a doctor.

Campylobacter infection. Transmission of *Campylobacter* is from food, mostly poultry, water, and sick individuals. The incubation period usually is two to five days.

Symptoms are diarrhea that can be bloody, fever, and abdominal pain. Diagnosis is made by culturing the bacteria. Therapy is antibiotics.

Cholera. Cholera is caused by bacteria, called *Vibrio cholerae.* Incubation period is one to three days.

The infection is caused by ingestion of contaminated water or food. Raw and undercooked shellfish is often the source.

Symptoms are large watery stools and vomiting that can lead to severe, life-threatening fluid loss.

Diagnosis is made by culturing the bacteria from the stool. Dehydration occurs very quickly.

Treatment is rehydration and antibiotics.

Parasites

Giardia. The disease spreads from person to person, from contaminated drinking water, or from pools. Incubation period is one to three weeks.

Giardia can cause long-lasting (chronic) or intermittent diarrhea. The stools are watery and foul-smelling.

Other symptoms are poor appetite and distention of the abdomen.

Treatment is a medication, metronidazole.

Ameba infection. The infection spreads from person to person. Incubation period is two to four weeks. Symptoms are watery or bloody diarrhea, abdominal cramps, and weight loss.

Treatment is drug therapy.

Cryptosporidiosis. Transmission of cryptosporidium occurs from contaminated drinking water and pools. Incubation period is three to fourteen days.

The most common symptom is watery diarrhea. But there can also be vomiting, abdominal cramps, and weight loss.

Usually, no specific treatment is necessary, but there is medicine for younger children.

Worms. Worms also can cause diarrhea.

The diagnosis of these diseases is made by checking the stool with the naked eye or under a microscope.

Treatment is drug therapy.

Bloody diarrhea, abdominal pain, vomiting. If a young child has severe abdominal pain, screams periodically, and is passing a small amount of bloody diarrhea with mucus and vomits, there is suspicion of an acute abdominal event called *intussusception.* That is a form of bowel obstruction, and it is an emergency. Go to the emergency room right away, or call 911. (See stomachache.)

Blood in the stool can be present for more benign reasons as well.

It can happen that blood gets into the stool from a rectal tear secondary to constipation or from a sore caused by a diaper rash. Older children can have bleeding from hemorrhoids. But in this case, there is no diarrhea, and the blood is only on the surface of the stool and not mixed in, unlike when the child has bloody diarrhea.

Other causes of diarrhea

Overeating

Food poisoning. Diarrhea and vomiting start two to six hours after the contaminated food is ingested. Symptoms are rapid onset of vomiting and diarrhea, maybe fever. The cause is contaminated food containing bacteria, viruses, and parasites. Diagnosis can be made from stool samples. Therapy depends on the cause. The child needs to drink plenty of fluids.

Lack of a digestive enzyme lactose (lactose intolerance). That can be congenital or transient.

Symptoms are diarrhea, abdominal cramps, and bloated stomach.

Diarrhea often causes temporary lactose intolerance. Therefore, it is important to stop milk and dairy products for a few days if your child has diarrhea.

Gluten intolerance (celiac disease). In celiac disease, there is a sensitivity to gluten. Foods containing gluten are wheat, rye, oats, barley. The gluten damages the surface of the small bowels, where food absorption is taking place.

Symptoms are diarrhea, weight loss, swollen abdomen (abdominal distention). The stools are shiny from the high fat content.

Anemia and vitamin deficiency can develop. Growth and weight gain are slow. The disease occurs more often in some families.

The diagnosis is made by laboratory tests, but it needs to be confirmed by endoscopy (a tube is placed to the mouth and moved down to the bowels under anesthesia) and biopsy (small piece of tissue is taken out and examined under microscope).

Treatment: the child needs to avoid foods that contain gluten, so needs to be on a gluten-free diet in order to grow and gain weight appropriately.

Antibiotics. Antibiotics also can cause diarrhea by decreasing the amount of protective bacteria in the bowels. A harmful bacteria, called *Clostridium difficile* (*C. diff.*) can grow, causing severe diarrhea, often with fever and abdominal pain.

The name of the disease caused by *C. diff* is called *pseudomembranous colitis.*

The diagnosis is made by laboratory tests from a stool sample and/or endoscopy and biopsy.

Treatment is medication, like metronidazole.

Proper use of antibiotics is important to prevent this infection. (Some parents want the doctor to prescribe antibiotics even if their child has a viral infection, in which case it does not help but can cause harm.)

Probiotics or eating yoghurt containing "good bacteria" (acidophilus, lactobacillus, etc.) during an antibiotic treatment helps to prevent diarrhea.

Inflammatory bowel disease like Crohn disease and ulcerative colitis can also cause diarrhea that can be bloody (see stomachache).

Diarrhea and vomiting

If the child has both symptoms together, he or she has gastroenteritis (infection, inflammation of the stomach and bowels).

The important thing is to be sure that the baby or child does not get dehydrated from fluid loss.

Babies get dehydrated easily. The more frequent the diarrhea and/or vomiting and the younger the baby is, the more likely dehydration develops (see dehydration).

If the baby or child has diarrhea more than four times and/or vomiting twice within twenty-four hours, he needs to see the doctor.

Treatment of diarrhea:

The first thing is to stop feeding. Sometimes after the baby has diarrhea or vomiting a few times, parents are worried that he or she is starving. So they continue to feed him or her, giving formula, and the result is more diarrhea and vomiting. On the other hand, if we temporarily stop feeding, the vomiting will stop, and the diarrhea will improve. However, we have to provide appropriate fluid intake. The lost water, sugar, and electrolytes need to be replenished. Pedialyte can be given for babies and young children. Pedialyte contains all the water, sugar, and electrolytes they need. Do not feed plain water to infants. For older children, Gatorade serves the same purpose. Babies and children with gastroenteritis need plenty of fluids, but start slowly. Give the liquid cold because that helps to stop the vomiting.

If there is no vomiting anymore and the diarrhea slows down, foods can be reinstituted slowly. Breastfeeding can be resumed. If the baby is on a milk-based formula, it is usually changed to soy or an elemental formula—like Nutramigen, Progestimil, or Alimentum—temporarily (as mentioned above, temporary lactose intolerance can develop secondary to diarrhea). Children usually can start to eat the so-called BRAT diet. That includes bananas, rice, applesauce, and toast. After two to three days, gradually go back to regular diet. Fried, heavy foods, milk, and dairy products should be the last ones reintroduced. It is important to follow the doctor's instructions because the baby cannot be without food too long, but with the introduction of food too soon, the diarrhea can get worse. Do not treat infants with antidiarrheal medications.

Prevention:

- The best prevention is good handwashing.
- Meat and poultry should be thoroughly cooked.
- Do not give your child raw or undercooked eggs.
- Powdered infant formulas are not sterile, so when reconstituting, boil the water. Be careful.
- Give your child only pasteurized milk and dairy products.
- Give your child only pasteurized juices.
- Do not give your child raw shellfish.
- Fruits and vegetables have to be rubbed and washed thoroughly several times with a strong stream of running water. Knives and containers used for raw meat should not be used to clean vegetables and fruits.
- Be sure that your child plays and swims in clean water, natural or pool.
- Prevent your child from playing with turtles to avoid salmonella infections.

Dehydration

Dehydration is caused by fluid loss, regardless of the cause.

Severe diarrhea and/or vomiting are the most common causes of dehydration.

However, high fever, rapid breathing, and decreased fluid intake also can cause dehydration or can make it more severe.

Increased urine output, like in diabetes mellitus and diabetes insipidus, can also cause dehydration. (See thirst, drinking large amount of fluids, urinating much.)

Symptoms:

- Weakness (the child might have problem walking).
- Weight loss.
- Sunken eyes.
- Dry coated tongue.
- Acetone smell in the breath.
- Apathy. That means that the child is inactive, does not want to play, is not interested in the surroundings, and only wants to sleep.

Decreased amount of urine, or no urination at all for eight to nine hours.

The soft spot (fontanelle) is sunken in babies.

If any of these symptoms are present, see the doctor. But if the child is apathetic or has no urine for eight to nine hours, go to the emergency room. However, if he or she is not responsive, call 911.

The younger the baby or child is and the more severe the symptoms are, the sooner medical help is necessary.

Dieting, extreme dieting, anorexia nervosa

Keep your child on a healthy, well-balanced diet. Give him much vegetables and fruits. Avoid extra salt and sugar, junk foods, and sugary drinks. Also, be sure that your child does not take dietary supplements (unless the doctor recommended), too much vitamins, and performance-enhancing substances because they can be harmful. If your adolescent is on a vegan diet, she needs vitamin supplements. Discuss it with her doctor. If your child needs to lose weight, try to achieve it gradually.

If a preadolescent girl keeps a vigorous diet, refuses food, and has a significant weight loss, she probably has an eating disorder called *anorexia nervosa*. In that case, the self-image is often distorted. She thinks that she is fat when she is not, so she wants to lose weight. She wants to eat less and only foods with low calories. Besides, she probably wants to do vigorous exercises to achieve her goal. Often the temperature, pulse rate, and blood pressure decrease. The condition can be so severe that hospitalization becomes necessary. Therefore, early intervention and close follow-up is important. Psychotherapy is often needed.

Dizziness

Dizziness is a sensation of losing balance.

The important question is whether the child feels uncertain, is losing balance, light-headed, or feels that the room is going around.

If the child feels that the room goes around, it is called *vertigo*. Vomiting often accompanies vertigo.

Causes of vertigo:

- Chronic middle ear infection, inner ear infection, or disturbance
- Head injury
- Migraine
- Neurologic diseases

Meniere disease is recurrent attacks of vertigo. It is rare in children.

Dizziness can also be caused by high or low blood pressure, low blood sugar, irregular heartbeats. Before fainting, the child feels dizzy as well.

If the child has dizziness, a checkup is necessary.

In case of *vertigo*, often an ear doctor (otolaryngologist) and/or a neurologist are consulted.

Down syndrome

Down syndrome is a genetic disorder. It is caused by a chromosomal abnormality (trisomy 21).

The child with Down syndrome has special features: short stature, short fingers, short neck, protruding tongue, upward slanting eyelids, skin fold at the inner corner of the eyes (epicanthus), and single crease in the palm. He also has decreased muscle tone, strength, and mental disability. Vision and hearing problem can be present as well.

The risk of having a child with Down syndrome increases with the advancing age of the mother.

The diagnosis can be made prenatally from amniotic fluid obtained by amniocenteses (see tests, procedures, surgeries).

Diagnosis is made after birth by the clinical features and chromosome analysis from a blood sample.

Complications can include heart disease, low thyroid hormone level (hypothyroidism), problems with the digestive system, sleep apnea, and spine problem (misalignment of the top vertebra-*atlantoaxial instability*.) A child with Down syndrome has a higher risk of leukemia.

Because of the possible neck problem, it is very important to have a neck x-ray before participating in sports.

There is no treatment for Down syndrome, but the complications can be treated.

Many children with Down syndrome need special education.

Early intervention is important.

Drooling

Common causes of drooling:

- Teething
- Spicy foods
- Chemicals (poisons)
- Difficulty swallowing: diseases of the esophagus, foreign body
- Ulcers in the mouth, like when the child has hand, foot and mouth disease
- Infections of the throat, tonsillitis, peritonsillar abscess, retropharyngeal abscess (see sore throat)
- Epiglottitis (see cough, respiratory problems, respiratory distress)
- Neurologic problems with developmental delay

Treatment depends on the cause.

Drowning

Drowning is a common cause of death in the US. Prevention of drowning is most important.

Babies and young children should not stay alone in the bathtub, not even for a second. Drain the bathtub right after you bathe your child.

Pools need to be fenced all around and have a gate that is self-closing. Be sure that your child cannot climb the fence, cannot reach the latches, and cannot get to the pool in any way.

Be sure that your teenager does not drink alcohol when swimming or boating. Have a pool alarm, but that does not substitute your watching eyes. Do not leave toys in the pool. Have a firm retractable pool cover, and close the pool and also the hot tub if not in use. Use drain covers so your child's hair is not sucked in. Do not leave water in inflatable pools.

Empty buckets after use. Keep the bathroom and toilet doors closed.

Do not let your child play on thin ice.

If your child cannot swim, an adult should be with him in the water all the time, and he should wear a life jacket. Children and adolescents also should wear life jackets when boating.

Teach your child to swim early on.

If a child has seizures, he cannot stay in the water alone.

After drowning, cardiopulmonary resuscitation (CPR) should be started, and call 911. Treating conditions that occur with drowning is necessary, like irregular heartbeats or arrhythmia, shock, seizure, and low temperature (hypothermia).

Dyslexia

Dyslexia is a learning disorder in reading.

It is characterized by difficulties recognizing words. Children with dyslexia have problem relating speech sounds to letters and words. They have problem understanding what they read, and it is difficult for them to recall it. They have difficulty understanding what was said and pronounce a new word. A child with dyslexia also has problem with spelling.

Because of the reading problem, a child with dyslexia can have difficulties with other subjects as well since reading is the basis of learning.

Dyslexia is usually recognized when the child starts school and has a problem learning reading. Generally, the teacher is the first who identifies the problem.

If your child has more difficulty with reading than other children of his age, see the doctor.

In that case, he needs an evaluation and treatment. Early intervention is important.

Treatment:

- Tutoring
- Classroom accommodation
- Individual education plan
- Emotional support and encouragement to prevent the development of low self-esteem and behavioral problems

The parent, the doctor, other health professionals, and the school need to work together.

Ear infection (otitis media)

Ear infection is common during infancy and childhood. The older the child gets, the frequency of ear infections decreases.

Acute ear infection. Acute ear infection often develops from an upper respiratory infection.

What is usually called ear infection is a middle ear infection (otitis media).

Symptoms: The baby becomes fussy, often crying or screaming mostly at night or when lying on the back. Fever often develops. Vomiting and diarrhea are common. The baby often has a runny nose, tags or pulls the ear, and it is painful to the touch. However, babies can have an ear infection without these symptoms.

Therefore, it is advisable to take the baby to the doctor if he or she has a lingering "cold" (upper respiratory infection). Also, if the baby does not act right, is not happy, does not eat or sleep well, a doctor's visit is a good idea.

Children complain of earache. Sometimes there is drainage from the ear canal that can be pus or bloody discharge. It means that the ear drum has a hole. It is perforated. It usually heals after several months, but regular follow-up is needed. If it does not heal for a long time, usually an ear doctor (otolaryngologist) is consulted, and maybe surgery is needed to cover the hole with a patch.

Ear infection can cause temporary hearing loss until the fluid in the middle ear is absorbed.

Chronic ear infection. Chronic ear infection can cause hearing loss.

Treatment of ear infections is often antibiotic, particularly for babies. Older children do not always need antibiotics, but then close follow-up is necessary.

Follow-up is always needed after an ear infection to be sure that it has resolved and the fluid behind the eardrum has gone.

If the middle ear fluid does not clear, the infection can recur because it is a good medium for bacteria to grow.

If the child has constant ear infection for a long time, or it frequently recurs, ear tube placement can be the solution and a last resort.

Ear infections can have complications, particularly if they have not been treated or have not been cured for a long time.

Complications: mastoiditis, cholesteatoma, meningitis (see below).

Mastoiditis

If a child developed mastoiditis, it means that the infection reached the bone behind the ear. There is soft swelling and redness behind the ear. If you noticed that, call the doctor right away. An otolaryngologist is usually involved in the child' s care.

Treatment: intravenous (IV) antibiotics, often surgery.

Cholesteatoma

After a long-lasting infection a soft mass can develop at the eardrum, that requires surgery.

Meningitis (infection of the membranes around the brain)

Symptoms are fever, vomiting, lethargy. That is an emergency, so go to the emergency room, or call 911. (See vomiting.)

Outer ear infection (otitis externa) or swimmer's ear. Swimmer's ear is an infection of the outer ear canal (external canal). It usually develops after swimming in a pool or natural water; therefore, it is more common in the summer.

It is usually caused by bacteria.

Symptoms are earache, pain when the earlobe is moved, and usually some white material is present in the ear canal. Middle ear infection also can develop from swimmer's ear.

The child needs to see the doctor.

Treatment is usually ear drops, sometimes antibiotics.

Since the infection is caused by water in the ear, be sure to keep the infected ear canal dry. Ear plugs can prevent swimmer's ear.

A foreign body in the ear canal or the use of a Q-tip, causing injury, can also contribute to the development of outer ear infection.

Foreign body in the ear canal can be suspected if there is a constant foul odor coming from the ear canal. (See foreign body.)

Emergencies

Call 911 in the following circumstances:

- If the airway is blocked, choking.
- If there is no breathing or if the breathing is very slow and the child is gasping for air.
- If there is no pulse, and the lips and face turn blue.

If any of these events happen, start cardiopulmonary resuscitation (CPR) immediately, and call 911. It is important that everybody learn CPR, particularly people who have or want children.

- If the child was drowning (see drowning).
- If the child has a severe injury.
- If the child has a severe burn, or inhalation injury from direct heat or steam (see burns).
- If the child is unconscious or lethargic (see neck pain: stiff neck).
- If the child has a seizure (see jerking and strange movements).
- If the child has respiratory distress, hard breathing, or the baby or child is gasping for air, the respiration is loud, and there is pulling in on the neck, below the Adam's apple, and/or under the rib cage (see cough, respiratory problems, respiratory distress).
- If the breathing is irregular or very slow and insufficient with occasional gasping and color change. (Babies can have irregular breathing during the first few weeks. If there are no other symptoms and it lasts only for twenty seconds and otherwise the baby is okay, that is normal.)
- If the child has signs of shock—altered mental status, cold sweat, and fast heart rate and breathing (see change of consciousness, fast breathing, cold sweat, shock).

- If there is a severe allergic reaction, swelling of the tongue, neck, loud and troubled breathing, or if the child feels that his throat is closing in (see allergic reaction).
- If you think that your child is so sick that any delay of medical help would harm him or her.

Go to the emergency room or call 911 in the following circumstances:

- If the child has a poisoning (see poisonings).
- If the child has an injury.
- If the child had the first seizure or the seizure lasted longer than five minutes.
- If the child has eye injury (see eye problems).
- If there is significant bleeding.
- If the child has a foreign body (see foreign bodies).
- If the child swallowed a battery (see foreign bodies).
- If the child behaves strangely, or if there is any change in mental status (see substance abuse).
- If the child had a concussion (see concussion).
- If the child has a strong throbbing headache (see headaches).
- If the child developed weakness of any extremities (see muscle weakness).
- If the child has difficulty breathing or loud breathing (see cough, respiratory problems, respiratory distress).
- If the child has severe vomiting (see vomiting).
- If the child has severe diarrhea (see diarrhea).
- If the child is dehydrated, and has no urine for eight to nine hours (see dehydration).
- If the child has severe abdominal pain (see stomachache).
- If the child has a testicular injury or pain and swelling of a testicle (testicular torsion).
- If the child got a human, animal, scorpion, snake, spider (black widow and brown recluse) bite or a bad jellyfish sting (see bites).

- If the child has swelling of the eyelids, lips, hands, or feet, or hives and itching (see allergic reaction).
- If the child has significant chest pain (see chest pain).
- If the child has a deep cut (see cuts: lacerations).
- If the child has joint pain and limping (see flat foot and other orthopedic problems).
- If the child cannot walk or is walking strangely by wobbling (see concussion).
- If the child's extremities are swollen, and/or painful and movements are limited (see broken bones: fractures).
- If the child has fever of 104 degrees Fahrenheit or above (see fever).
- If you think that your child is so sick that he or she needs immediate medical attention.

If any of the above conditions are severe, call 911.

In case of severe injury, it is very important not to move the child and not to sit or stand him or her up.

It is best to leave the child on the ground until the ambulance arrives.

Head trauma often causes neck injury, so do not move the head. If an injured head or neck is moved, there is a risk of spinal cord injury.

In case of bleeding, put pressure on the wound, preferably with sterile gauze or clean cloth. If they are not available and the bleeding is heavy, put pressure on the wound with your fingers to stop the bleeding.

Bleeding of the scalp from a cut can be hidden by the hair, so you need to look for it.

In case of head injury, the child often has a concussion.

Important questions:

- Has the child lost consciousness?
- Does the child remember what happened? Who talked to him or her first after passing out, and what did he say?

- Was there any vomiting?
- Was the child able to walk? Was the walking normal as usual, or was it wobbly?
- Was the child dizzy?
- Does the child have a headache?
- Was the vision okay after the trauma?
- Was the hearing okay after the injury?

It is very important not to resume physical and mental activity after a concussion. A concussion should be taken seriously to avoid serious consequences.

The child needs to see a doctor as soon as possible. A neurologist or sports medicine doctor is often involved with the child's care. The instructions of the doctor should be strictly followed, including the time frame going back to school and sports. (See concussion.)

Eye problems

Tearing and mucus in the eye. Tearing and mucus in the eye is commonly caused by eye disease, eye injury, and a foreign body.

However, tearing can be caused by other diseases too, like upper respiratory infection (URI), or some infectious diseases, like measles.

Pink eye (conjunctivitis). Pink eye is most commonly caused by viruses, bacteria, and allergies. But there are other significant causes as well, like uveitis (see later in this chapter).

Inward-turning eyelashes also can cause irritation of the eyes. They need to be removed by an eye doctor.

Symptoms of pink eye are different degrees of redness, discharge, often yellow or green. Tearful, itchy eyes, and discomfort are common.

Pink eye is contagious; therefore, good handwashing is imperative.

If your child has pink eyes, he or she needs to stay home and see the doctor.

Treatment is eye drops or ointment.

Newborns and babies can have mucus in the eyes by having pink eyes. But if only a small amount of mucus is present in the eye, wipe it off with slightly warm water. Use a piece of gauze. If the baby's eye is not red but always tearing or has mucus and affects only one eye, *obstruction of the tear duct* is likely.

Treatment of tear duct obstruction:

- See the doctor.
- Massage of the tear point (that is located at the inner corner of the eye) sometimes solves the problem.
- Antibiotic drops or ointment can be necessary.
- If the condition does not improve by the massage, an eye doctor (ophthalmologist) needs to be consulted, who can place a small probe into the tear duct to open the blockage.

In case of tear duct obstruction, the *tear sac can get infected (dacryocystitis).*

The symptoms are redness, warmth, tenderness, and swelling at the corner of the eye. When the tear point is pressed, pus comes out. Again, the tear point is located at the corner of the eye.

Treatment: antibiotics.

Eye injuries. If the pink eye affects only one eye, it can raise the suspicion of trauma or foreign body. (However, pink eye can start on one eye and spread to the other one). The clinical picture is similar, so ask your child if he has hurt his eye or feels that anything has gotten into his eye.

Trauma, foreign bodies, and chemical burns can injure the eyes. A severely injured eye can endanger the other eye too.

The symptoms are pain, continuous tearing, sensitivity to light (photosensitivity). The child does not want to open his eyes. Blurry vision or impaired vision can be present as well. In the case of a *foreign body*, there is a sensation that something is in the eye. Eyelashes are often the foreign bodies. In that case, you can try to wash it out with water. Often the tears get rid of the eyelash.

If a chemical gets into the eye, wash it out with running water or syringe for at least ten minutes.

All eye injuries and foreign bodies need urgent medical attention, so go to the emergency room, or call 911 right away.

Pink eye caused by allergies is called *allergic or vernal conjunctivitis.*

Treatment is antihistamine eye drops like Patanol, Pataday, Zaditor.

Chronic inflammation of the eyelid margin (blepharitis). Chronic reddening and itching of the eyelid margin is characteristic. Often fine scales can be seen at the base of eyelashes. Blepharitis can be caused by infection or irritation of the skin (dermatitis). Treatment is warm soaking and, if needed, antibiotic ointment. When you use warm soaking, put a piece of gauze in warm water, then squeeze the water out. Place the gauze on the eyelids for five minutes. When the gauze is not warm anymore, put it back into the warm water. Do the soaking four times a day. Be sure that the water is not too hot.

Uveitis. Uveitis is inflammation in the eye. It can be caused by infection or systemic disease, like Kawasaki disease (see heart problems) or juvenile rheumatoid arthritis.

Symptoms of uveitis are pink eye, pain, tearing, sensitivity to light.

Eye doctor (ophthalmologist) needs to be involved in the child's care.

Treatment is usually steroid eye drops. However, even if you happen to have steroid eye drops at home, never use them without the instruction of the doctor. It can be harmful if it is used for the wrong reason.

Keratitis and corneal ulcer. Cornea is a transparent layer covering the pupil and the colorful part of the eye (iris).

Keratitis is the inflammation of the cornea.

Ulcers on the cornea can develop from infection caused by the herpes virus or other infections after injury.

Both conditions are very painful.

Ophthalmologists are treating these conditions.

Drooping of the upper eyelid (ptosis). Ptosis is the drooping of the upper eyelid. It can be present from birth or can develop later. If it exists from birth and covers a large portion of the pupil, it can interfere with the development of vision. It needs to be checked by an eye doctor (ophthalmologist), and if it is significant, surgery might be necessary.

Cross eye (strabismus). If the child has a cross-eye, the eyes deviate. It is usually caused by an imbalance of the eye muscles.

In the first five months, babies do not have coordinated eye movements, so they can have cross-eye.

However, if you see that your baby has a cross-eye after five to six months of age, show it to the doctor.

It is also useful to take pictures.

Some babies and children have large nasal bridge that can give the impression of cross-eye, when in fact that is not the case. Anyway, it needs to be checked out.

Children do not use the eye that deviates, so *lazy eye (amblyopia)* can develop. Lazy eye significantly impairs vision; therefore, early detection and treatment is most important.

Parents and pediatricians can suspect lazy eye, but consultation with an ophthalmologist is needed to make the diagnosis and treat the condition.

Treatment is usually patching of the affected eye, glasses, or, if no improvement, surgery.

Double vision (diplopia). If a young child squints, holds one of his eyes, or has an abnormal head position, like tilting the head, double vision is suspected. The origin of double vision can be in the eye, like cross-eye (strabismus), or in the central nervous system (brain). Injury of the bone around the eye (orbit) also can cause double vision. Therefore, the child urgently needs to see the doctor, who will decide whether he or she needs to see an eye doctor, a neurologist, or both. In case of injury to the orbit, an ENT (ear, nose, throat) doctor is involved in the child's care.

Repetitive jerking of the eyes (nystagmus). Nystagmus is always considered to be a serious symptom. Therefore, the child urgently needs to see the doctor to get a full evaluation. Usually an ophthalmologist and a neurologist are involved in the child's care.

Cataract. Cataract is clouding (opacity) of the lens in the eye.

Cataracts can be present at birth (congenital cataract) or develop later.

Frequent causes of cataracts:

- Infections of the mother
- Certain metabolic disorders, like galactosemia (see breastfeeding)

- Eye trauma
- Chemical burn
- Some eye diseases
- Long-term use of steroids
- Congenital rubella or varicella

Cataracts can affect vision.

Treatment: If the lens becomes opaque, surgery is needed. An eye doctor (ophthalmologist) takes care of the child with cataract.

Glaucoma. Glaucoma means increased pressure inside the eye (intraocular pressure). It can involve one or both eyes. The increased pressure can damage the optic nerve. A child can be born with glaucoma, but injury of the eye can cause it as well.

Treatment is conducted by an ophthalmologist.

Antiglaucoma medications often control the pressure in the eye, but sometimes surgery is necessary.

Nearsightedness (myopia), farsightedness (hyperopia). If the child cannot see an object in the distance or is holding a book close to the eye, nearsightedness is suspected.

The opposite is farsightedness, when the child cannot see objects that are too close. In this case, he or she holds the book very far from the eye.

Both conditions are treated by eye doctors with corrective lenses (glasses).

Astigmatism. Astigmatism is a refractive error. It is a type of vision problem caused by an irregular curvature of the cornea (the front surface of the eye that is clear) or the lens. It causes distorted or blurry vision.

Treatment is eyeglasses.

Stye (Hordeolum). If the child has a bump on the eyelid, that is often a stye or sometimes chalazion (see below). In case of a stye, the bump is red and tender, and frequently, a white or yellow point is seen in the area. Stye is the infection of the glands of the eyelid.

Treatment is frequently changed warm compresses. Sometimes also a local antibiotic is needed.

Chalazion. Chalazion is a small painless lump on the upper or lower eyelid, but can be painful when developing from a stye.

Treatment is initially warm soaks and antibiotic ointment.

If there is no improvement, surgery may be necessary.

Failure to thrive (FTT)

Failure to thrive means that the weight and height of a baby or child is much less than of others of the same age and sex. So the weight and height is less than 3 percentile on the growth chart. Usually, first the weight lags behind, then the height follows.

Many things can cause failure to thrive, so it is important to find the causes.

FTT can be caused by the following:

- Poor nutrition.
- Trouble swallowing.
- Frequent vomiting (pyloric stenosis, gastroesophageal reflux).
- Inappropriate absorption of the nutrients from the bowels. (Food malabsorption, celiac disease.)
- The child has been losing more calories than he or she took in (overactive thyroid gland or hyperthyroidism, diabetes mellitus).
- There are other causes too, like chronic diseases, including heart, kidney, bowel, liver disease, chronic infectious diseases, cystic fibrosis, parasites.
- Developmental delays, genetic diseases and disorders.
- Other causes are psychological, maternal depression, and lack of resources. See details below.

Important questions and causes of failure to thrive (FTT):

- What was the baby's gestational age and birth weight? Premature babies, particularly those with very small birth weight, are behind with weight and height in the first year, but after that, they usually catch up.
- How many times is the baby fed? How much does he or she eat? If the breast milk is not enough, the baby needs formula supplement. If the baby is formula-fed, how does

mom prepare the formula (if it needs to be mixed)? Because if the formula is too diluted, it does not provide enough calories for the baby to gain weight. Prepare according to directions.

- How many times does the child eat, and how much? It is best to write a diary about the child's diet for at least two weeks, including the amounts, and take it to the doctor for the checkup.

- Is the baby's sucking and swallowing normal? If not, that can lead to FTT. Tongue tie (tight frenulum of the tongue called ankyloglossia), for example, can cause breastfeeding problems. It can require surgery to release the tongue.

- Has the baby or child been vomiting? Chronic vomiting as in case of gastroesophageal reflux (GE reflux) or gastroesophageal reflux disease (GERD) can cause FTT (see vomiting).

- Pyloric stenosis can cause FTT (see vomiting).

- Has the baby or child been having any diarrhea? Is there any blood or mucus in the stool? Is the color normal? Is there any foul smell? Are the stools shiny? In case of chronic diarrhea, the nutrients obtained from the food do not absorb from the bowels to the blood as normally (malabsorption). An example is lactose intolerance (see diarrhea). Chronic diarrhea can be caused by parasites, like giardia, as well. Gluten sensitivity as in celiac disease (see stomachache) or pancreas insufficiency like in cystic fibrosis (see cough, respiratory problems, respiratory distress) can cause chronic diarrhea and FTT as well. Another example is inflammatory bowel disease like Crohn's disease and ulcerative colitis (see stomachache).

- Is the urination okay? Is the frequency and the amount normal? If the urine production is too much (polyuria), it can be caused by kidney problems, like urinary tract infection, renal tubular acidosis (the acid production in the urine by the kidneys is impaired), chronic renal failure. Again, chronic diseases can cause FTT.

- Has the child been having a chronic cough? Tuberculosis and cystic fibrosis also can cause FTT. (See cough, respiratory problems, respiratory distress.)
- Insulin deficit with high blood sugar (diabetes mellitus) can cause increased amounts of urine and weight loss.
- Decreased secretion of the antidiuretic hormone (diabetes insipidus) can cause the same. (See thirst, drinking large amount of fluids and urinating much.)
- Kidney (renal) failure.
- If the thyroid gland is overworking (hyperthyroidism), the child burns more calories than he or she takes in, so FTT can be the consequence.
- Congenital heart disease can lead to FTT because the calorie intake is not appropriate.
- Infectious diseases, like human immunodeficiency virus (HIV) can cause FTT.
- Chronic hepatitis can cause FTT.
- Children with worms may not absorb enough nutrients, so develop FTT.

The diagnosis of failure to thrive is made by the history, physical exam, laboratory tests, and/or x-ray, depending on the cause.

Treatment is diet correction and treating the cause.

Fainting

Fainting is a sudden, temporary loss of consciousness.

The child feels dizzy before fainting, loses consciousness, falls to the ground. Recovery is usually quick.

A child also can faint if he or she cannot catch air because of choking, breath-holding spell (temper tantrum), fast and deep breathing hyperventilation (anxiety attack), whooping cough, or, rarely, asthma.

Some children faint when they stand up suddenly, and their *blood pressure drops (orthostatic hypotension)*.

These children need to get up slowly, avoid standing for a long time, particularly in a crowd and hot weather.

Some children faint when they get shot, by the same mechanism.

Heart problems like arrhythmia also can cause fainting.

If your child fainted or almost fainted, he or she needs to see the doctor.

Try to prevent injury by catching the child before falling. If you see that the child will faint, she becomes very pale, hold her, and gently let her go to the ground. Do not move the child, keep the head to the side to prevent aspiration, and lift the legs up.

Fever

Elevated body temperature is most often caused by infection and inflammation. But there are other causes as well. For example, if your baby or child is overheated (heat exhaustion), he can have fever. Vaccines can cause fever as well.

There is some confusion about taking the temperature and evaluating fever.

There are different ways to take temperature: oral, under the arm (axillary), rectal, ear, and skin.

Rectal temperature is often taken on babies. Before you take a rectal temperature, put a little KY jelly or an ointment to the tip of the thermometer. Then push it to the rectum gently, and hold the cheeks of the bottom together until it is done.

Under-the-arm temperature can be taken at any age, including newborns. Best is to use a digital thermometer. If you have a baby or young child, hold his or her arm to be sure that the thermometer does not move.

For taking oral temperature, the child has to be old enough to keep the thermometer under the tongue.

When taking temperature with an ear thermometer, you place it to the ear with the tip that is disposable.

Skin thermometers measure the temperature of the forehead.

Digital thermometers are commonly used because they are accurate, clean (you can change the tip), and it can be used to measure oral, axillary, and rectal temperature. When the reading of the temperature is ready, you hear a beep.

The use of mercury thermometers is not advisable. They are accurate but can break, potentially causing injury or poisoning.

The temperature can be measured by two different scales: Fahrenheit (F) and Celsius (C).

Degrees of Fahrenheit are most commonly used in the USA in general, but hospitals often use the degrees of Celsius.

These are the conversions of some important degrees:

Degrees in Fahrenheit (F) Degrees in Celsius (C)

98.6 degrees F = 37 degrees C
99.4 degrees F = 37.4 degrees C
99.7 degrees F = 37.6 degrees C
100.1 degrees F = 37.8 degrees C
100.4 degrees F = 38 degrees C
101 degrees F = 38.3 degrees C
102.2 degrees F = 39 degrees C
102.6 degrees F = 39.2 degrees C
103.3 degrees F = 39.6 degrees C
104 degrees F = 40 degrees C
105 degrees F = 40.6 degrees C
105.8 degrees F = 41 degrees C

The range of normal temperature is between 97.6 and 99.6 degrees Fahrenheit or 36 and 37.4 degrees Celsius.

Body temperature is usually lowest in the morning and highest in the evening, around 6:00 p.m.

As mentioned above, there is a confusion about evaluating temperatures because the normal oral, axillary, and rectal temperatures are slightly different. The temperature under the arm is the lowest, and the rectal temperature is the highest.

The difference between axillary and rectal temperature is about 1 degree Fahrenheit. Because of the difference, parents sometimes mistakenly add 1 degree to the measured axillary temperature. That can make the difference between normal temperature and fever. If the measured temperature, for example, is 99.4 degrees Fahrenheit, which is normal, but the parent adds 1 degree to it, then the child would have a fever of 100.4 degrees Fahrenheit.

Therefore, the best way is to tell the doctor the measured temperature, how it was taken, and what kind of thermometer was used.

Parents sometimes say that the child had a fever, but they did not take the temperature but gave him or her Tylenol. It is more helpful, however, if the doctor knows what the temperature actually was.

If the child has fever, it is best to take the temperature three times a day, including at 6:00 p.m. and any time you think he or she might have fever.

Fever can cause dehydration, so be sure that your child gets plenty of fluids.

Some children have seizures from high fever. If your child is one of them, after the first seizure, anytime he has the slightest elevation of temperature, or looks like he is getting sick, start a fever reducer like ibuprofen or Tylenol. Also, seizure precautions are necessary (see jerking and strange movements). If the child has the first seizure, call 911.

Treatment of fever is acetaminophen (Tylenol) or ibuprofen (Motrin, Advil).

Sometimes parents complain that even after they gave Tylenol to the child, the fever continues.

Tylenol does not necessarily take the temperature down to normal, but it decreases the fever. If, let's say, the fever was 103 degrees Fahrenheit, and the Tylenol brought it down to 101 degrees Fahrenheit, that is all you need, unless there is a history of seizure.

If the fever is continuously high and neither the acetaminophen nor the ibuprofen broke it, you can alternate the two. So you can give one, then the other every four hours. But acetaminophen cannot be given more often than every four hours and cannot be given more than five times during a twenty-four-hour period.

Similarly, ibuprofen cannot be given more often than every six hours and cannot be given more than four times over twenty-four hours.

If the child has a fever, it is important to remove most of his clothes. Some parents are hesitant to do that, but it helps to reduce the fever.

If the fever remains high, 103.5–104 degrees Fahrenheit, you can give a sponge bath. You place your child in the bathtub, and splash him or her with lukewarm water, including the head. After five to ten minutes, dry your child, and check the temperature. If it is lower than 102 degrees F, you can stop the sponge bath. If the fever is still high, continue the sponge bath. If a bathtub is not available, you can wrap the child in wet sheets and change it frequently so it is always wet and not warm.

It is important not to give acetaminophen or ibuprofen more than a few days, unless the doctor has instructed you to do so. Both medications can cause serious side effects if overused (see poisoning). Use these medications only if it is really necessary. Sometimes parents use them even if the child only has a cold but feels okay and has no fever or pain.

Sometimes parents ask whether they can give acetaminophen or ibuprofen along with antibiotic or cold medicine. They can be used at the same time as the antibiotic, but be sure that the cold medicine does not contain acetaminophen or ibuprofen. Otherwise the child gets a double dose.

Take your child to the doctor in case of the following:

- If the fever is high.
- If the fever lasts longer than a day.
- If there are other symptoms besides fever and slight cold.
- If your baby has a fever. Any baby with a fever needs medical attention the same day the fever started.

Keep your child at home with fever, and he or she can only return to school if there is no fever for twenty-four hours.

It is very important to know that if a baby has a fever of 100 degrees Fahrenheit or higher in the first two to three months of life, urgent medical attention is necessary. So take your baby to the emergency room. In those first few months, often there are no other symptoms of a disease but fever. Also, infections can spread faster when the baby is so young.

Parents often think that if their child has no fever, he or she is not sick. But there are other symptoms equally or even more serious than fever, like vomiting and lethargy.

Important questions:

- When did the fever start, and how high was it?
- Is the child alert?
- Is there any lethargy? (Parents sometimes think that the child is lethargic if he or she is tired and not as active as usual. Doctors think that the child is lethargic if he or she is not responding or only responding for a short time, like for a few seconds or a minute, before falling back to sleep again.)
- How does the child behave? Does he or she act as usual, or is she weak, tired, sleepy, or irritable?
- How is the breathing? Is it normal or fast and labored or slow and irregular? Is the breathing noisy?
- Does the child have a cough, runny nose, or nasal congestion?
- Has the child had any vomiting?
- Has the child had any diarrhea?
- Does the child have a rash?
- Does the child have any pain or ache?
- Has the urination been okay? Are there any complaints with urination, like painful frequent urination and/or a weak urine stream?
- Are there any sores, bites, redness, or swelling?
- Does he walk okay?

Fever with other symptoms

Fever and cough. Fever and cough are common symptoms. These two symptoms most commonly occur if the child has a cold or upper respiratory infection (URI) caused by a virus. It is often accompanied by a runny nose, pink eye, and sore throat.

But fever and cough also can indicate bronchitis (inflammation of the tubes in the lung), bronchiolitis (inflammation of the small tubes in the lung), or pneumonia (infection of the lung) (see cough, respiratory problems, respiratory distress).

However, children can have bronchitis, bronchiolitis, and even pneumonia without fever.

Fast and/or hard breathing also can be present. If that is the case, urgent medical attention is needed. With all of the above conditions, the child needs to see the doctor. However, if the breathing is heavy, go to the emergency room, or call 911.

Fever and rash. Many contagious diseases appear with fever and rash, like chickenpox, measles, rubella, roseola, scarlet fever (see infectious diseases of childhood). Many other viral illnesses come with a rash too, and so is Kawasaki disease and Rocky Mountain spotted fever.

Kawasaki disease. This can be suspected if the high fever lasts longer than five days and the child is younger than five years.

Other symptoms are often rash, pink eye, red cracked lips, bright-red tongue, and enlarged lymph nodes.

The most important complication of Kawasaki disease is local bulging (aneurysm) in the so-called coronary arteries. The injury of the heart muscle can be the consequence since these arteries supply the heart with blood. The aneurysm is diagnosed by echocardiogram (echo). That is a sonogram of the heart.

Treatment is immune globulin administration into a vein (IV), aspirin, and steroids.

Rocky Mountain spotted fever (RMSF). This is a severe disease caused by a germ called *Rickettsia*. It presents with fever and rash.

RMSF occurs mostly in the South Atlantic, Southeastern, and Central US (not common in the Rocky Mountain area) mostly from April to September.

It is transmitted to people by tick bites.

Incubation period is about one week.

Symptoms are fever, muscle pain, headache, sensitivity to light, vomiting, often diarrhea. A rash develops with small red spots and bumps. It starts at the wrists and ankles, then appears on the palms and soles, then on the trunk. Rash with *petechiae* (see below) can develop later and indicate severe disease. Neurologic, heart, lung, kidney problems, and even shock (see change of consciousness, fast breathing, cold sweat) can develop.

History of a tick bite and early recognition of the disease is important.

The diagnosis is made by a blood test.

Treatment is antibiotics.

If your child has fever and rash, the doctor needs to be consulted.

So-called petechiae also look like a rash. But they are blood spots on the skin and look like pinpoint-size dark-red spots. If you press on these spots, they do not change, while a regular rash seems to fade under pressure.

Fever and petechiae. This usually indicates severe disease.

In case of *meningitis* (see vomiting) caused by a bacteria called meningococcus, the baby or child also has petechiae but fever, vomiting, and lethargy as well.

So if your child has fever and petechiae, go to the emergency room. But if he or she is also lethargic, call 911.

Petechiae are also present in *Henoch-Schönlein purpura*. Other symptoms are joint pain and stomachache.

Complication is kidney disease.

Treatment is steroid, rest, adequate fluid intake, and pain medications like Tylenol or ibuprofen. If the child has kidney disease, do not use ibuprofen, unless the doctor recommended.

Fever and vomiting. Many diseases can cause fever and vomiting. That is particularly true for infants since they can have vomiting with any disease, including ear infection.

Fever, vomiting, and abdominal pain. These three symptoms can indicate a problem in the abdomen like appendicitis. In case of *appendicitis,* the pain is usually on the right side of the lower abdomen. However, the pain also can be located at the navel. If your child has these symptoms, urgent medical attention is needed. Go to the emergency room.

Other less serious diseases, like strep throat, can cause the symptoms above as well.

Fever, vomiting, and abdominal pain also can indicate *urinary tract infection* (UTI). But in that case, other symptoms, like frequent painful, burning urination and bedwetting of a toilet-trained child, are often present as well. In younger children who cannot complain about pain, certain signs can raise the suspicion of UTI.

If the child refuses to go to the bathroom, if he or she bends over and holds the lower abdomen, or if she wets her pants or has frequent urination, UTI is suspected.

Fever and diarrhea. These are common symptoms of gastroenteritis (infection of the stomach and bowels). Vomiting is also common.

It is important to keep your child well hydrated. (See diarrhea.)

Fever, vomiting, lethargy. These symptoms can indicate infection of the central nervous system (brain), like meningitis. Urgent medical attention is necessary. Go to the emergency room, or call 911. (See vomiting.)

Fever and swollen nodes. Sore throat and infection of the tonsils (tonsillitis) often cause fever and swollen lymph nodes, most often on the neck.

If the child takes an antibiotic for those illnesses and the fever continues over two days, mononucleosis (mono), a viral disease, is suspected (see mononucleosis).

The symptoms of cat scratch disease are also fever and swollen nodes (see cat scratch disease).

Other viral illnesses also can cause enlarged lymph nodes. In case of rubella (a contagious disease caused by a virus), there are enlarged lymph nodes at the back of the head. (See infectious diseases of childhood.)

Sores and bites can cause the swelling of local lymph nodes and fever.

Fever of unknown origin (FUO). When a child has fever, the doctor asks about complaints, symptoms, and examines him or her. Most of the time, the doctor can make the diagnosis and initiate treatment. Therefore, it is frustrating to parents if that is not the case. If the only symptom is fever for two weeks or longer, and the physical exam, laboratory, and other tests are normal, the diagnosis is fever of unknown origin. In that case, follow-up is needed, and often the laboratory tests need to be repeated.

Flatfoot and other orthopedic problems

- Flat foot
- Toeing in
- Hip dysplasia
- Bowleg
- Dislocations
- Knock-knee
- Perthes disease
- Slipped capital femoral epiphysis
- Nursemaid's elbow
- Spine problems: curvature of the spine—scoliosis, kypnosis, lordosis, spondylolysis, spondylolisthesis ankylosing spondylitis, herniated disc, tumors
- Osgood-Schlatter disease
- Heel pain (Sever's apophysitis)
- Joint pain
- Limping
- Osteochondritis dissecans
- Osteomyelitis

Flatfoot. Flatfoot is a common condition. It means that the child's feet do not have a normal arch. During infancy and in the first six years of life, everybody has flat feet. Most flat feet do not cause problems. If the flatfoot is flexible, the foot becomes normal when the child is on tiptoe. If it is not flexible, then the flatfoot is more severe and can cause leg pain.

Treatment:

- Walking barefoot on grass is good for flatfoot.
- Select the type of shoes for your child that has an arch.
- If the flat foot is more prominent or causing complaint, inserts in the shoe can help. If the flat foot is severe, your

child's doctor will refer you to an orthopedic specialist or a foot doctor (podiatrist).

- It is a common question what kind of shoes a young child should wear. The good shoe is soft, flexible, and not tight. While walking barefoot is advantageous, be sure that your child has a shoe with a strong sole when walking on concrete.

Toeing in (pigeon toe)—metatarsus adductus. Toeing in is a condition when different parts of the leg and foot (the foot, the great toe, the ankle, the lower leg, the thigh bone) turn inward.

When the lower leg, the tibia, turns inward, it is called *tibial torsion.* If the thigh bone, the femur, turns inward, it is called *femoral anteversion.* Toeing in often makes parents worry. However, toeing in is usually a positional and not structural problem, and children usually grow out of it.

But if the inward position of the foot is rigid and the foot is curved and cannot be corrected at all, the child has *clubfoot (talipes equinovarus). Clubfoot* is usually present at birth.

Early diagnosis and orthopedic consultation is important.

Treatment: Multiple casting of the foot can correct clubfoot. If that is unsuccessful, surgery is necessary.

Hip dysplasia. The hip joint is a socket, and the head of the thigh bone (femur) is enclosed in it.

Congenital dysplasia of the hip is a condition when the hip socket does not fully cover the head of the thigh bone, and there is a tendency of the head of the thigh bone to come out from the hip socket.

Sometimes the head is out of the socket at birth, dislocated. It can be on one side or both.

It is more common in girls and in some families. Cesarean section and breech presentation (the fetus presents buttocks or feet first) increases the likelihood that the baby will have hip dysplasia.

Suspicion is raised by clinical signs, like hip click or if the hip is too loose or too tight. Also if there is a difference of the creases of the thighs and buttocks when the two sides are compared.

A likely clinical diagnosis is made by the doctor who checks the newborn, or during checkups throughout the first year.

The diagnosis is made by hip sonogram or by x-ray.

Early diagnosis is important.

Treatment:

- Consultation with an orthopedic specialist is necessary.
- A harness is most commonly used and highly successful. Pavlik harness is a soft brace that holds the head of the thigh bone in the hip socket. It keeps the legs apart and helps the development of the hip.
- If it does not resolve the problem, surgery can be necessary.

Bowleg. Bowleg is the curving of the leg, and it is normal in the first two years. The child can outgrow it even up to eight years of age.

Rickets caused by vitamin D deficiency can cause bowleg. The diagnosis is made by lab tests and/or x-ray. The treatment is a vitamin D supplement (see vitamins). A severe form of bowleg is called *Blount's disease.* The diagnosis is made by a physical exam and x-ray. Orthopedic consultation is needed.

Dislocations. Dislocation is an injury to a joint. The ends of the bones are forced from their normal position.

Symptoms: the joint is deformed, swollen, painful, immovable.

Therapy: Urgent medical attention is needed. Use crutches. Go to the emergency room. Usually an orthopedic surgeon participates in the child's care to place the bones back into normal position.

Fractures (see broken bones)

Heel pain (Sever's apophysitis)

Heel pain is most common in preadolescent boys playing sports. There is a focal tenderness of the heel. Treatment is heel cups or cushions and rest.

The shoes should provide adequate cushioning. If there is no improvement, see the doctor, and he might refer your child to an orthopedic specialist.

Knock knee (Genu valgum). In this condition, the legs are not straight, the knees are closer to each other, and the ankles are further from each other. It usually gets better with time.

If the condition is getting worse or persists after eight years of age, see the doctor.

Osgood-Schlatter disease. This is a common condition caused by overuse of the knee, usually from playing sports. A bump and swelling develops on the shinbone (tibia) just below the knee.

The child often complains of knee pain in the same area.

It often resolves with time.

Treatment:

- RICE: rest, ice, compression, and elevation (see muscle pain)
- Activities should be restricted
- Icing the painful area
- Anti-inflammatory medication like ibuprofen
- Knee pad or elastic wrap
- Physical therapy

Pain in the thigh or knee and limping. Knee pain often originates in the hip. Two diseases causing thigh or knee pain and limping are Perthes disease and slipped capital femoral epiphysis (see below).

Perthes disease. In this disease, there is interruption of the blood supply of the head of the thigh bone (femur). Consequently, the head will be deformed.

It occurs usually at two to twelve years of age.

Symptoms are thigh or knee pain and limping. There is a mild restriction of hip movements.

Diagnosis is made by x-ray or bone scan.

Consultation with an orthopedic surgeon is necessary.

Treatment: Rest is important. The child should be non-weight-bearing, using crutches.

Treatment depends on the severity of the condition. If the bone damage *is* significant, surgery is necessary.

Slipped capital femoral epiphysis. In this condition, there is a displacement of the head of the thigh bone. It usually occurs during adolescence and more commonly if the child is overweight.

Symptoms are thigh or knee pain, pain with hip motion, painful and difficult walking, and limping.

The diagnosis is made by x-ray.

Orthopedic consultation is necessary.

Treatment: rest, crutches, surgery.

Nursemaid's elbow. This condition occurs when a young child is pulled or lifted by the hand.

Symptoms: pain in the arm, and the child cannot move or bend the arm.

Treatment: Urgent medical attention is needed. The doctor repositions the child's arm. That is a simple treatment, and the pain stops at once.

For prevention, be sure that you and everybody else lift your child holding him or her under the armpit, not by the hand and not pulling the hand.

Spine problems

Curvature of the spine (scoliosis). Curvature of the spine can be present at birth (rarely) or can develop later on. Most commonly, scoliosis develops during adolescence, and it is called idiopathic scoliosis because the cause is unknown.

Scoliosis usually gets worse during the time of growth spurts; therefore, that is the most important time to look for it, and if it is present, check on it regularly. Therefore, checkups are so important in the time of adolescence.

When the doctor checks for scoliosis, the child will face the doctor and bend over. In case of scoliosis, there is a difference between the two sides of the back. If it is severe, it can be a hump there.

The diagnosis is made by a physical exam and x-ray.

Scoliosis needs to be followed closely. If it is getting worse or severe, an orthopedic surgeon needs to be consulted.

Treatment: spine brace or surgery if necessary.

With the above conditions, the child needs to see the doctor or an orthopedic specialist.

Kyphosis. Kyphosis is a forward curve of the upper back.

It can be secondary to bad posture (flexible kyphosis) or can be caused by a disease like Scheuermann disease, when the curve is rigid. That is a deformity of the spine.

Kyphosis can be congenital, or develops later.

Symptoms: the child can have a hump, back pain, and stiffness. Though a child with mild kyphosis may not have symptoms.

Diagnosis is made by physical exam and X ray. Sometimes MRI or CT scan is used as well.

When checking the child's back, it is best to look at it from the side.

Treatment depends on severity:

- Observation of the curve.
- Physical therapy.

- Back brace.
- Surgery if necessary.

Lordosis. When the spine curves too far inward, the child has lordosis (swayback).

Lordosis can affect the child's posture, but most of the time lordosis does not cause any symptoms.

Diagnosis and treatment are similar to kyphosis.

Defect of the spine (spondylolysis) (see back pain)

Spondylolysis. Sondylolysis is a stress fracture of the spine (vertebra). There is a small crack between two vertebras. Children playing contact sports are more prone to get this fracture.

It causes back pain.

Slippage of the vertebra can develop as well.

Diagnosis is made with physical exam, X ray, MRI, CT scan.

Treatment: rest, medications, corticosterioids, physical theraphy, bracing, and surgery if necessary.

Spondylolisthesis. Spondylolisthesis is a condition when the vertebra slips out of place.

Symptoms are back pain and stiffness. Problem walking, numbness, and weakness of the foot can be present as well.

Diagnosis is made by physical exam and X ray. Sometimes MRI, CT scan, or bone scan are needed.

Treatment: rest, medications, bracing, and surgery if necessary.

Ankylosing spondylitis (see back pain)

Herniated disc (see back pain)

Tumors (see back pain)

All of the conditions above are treated by orthopedic surgeons.

Limping. Limping is an important symptom.

It can be caused by the following:

- Injury of the bone (fracture), joint, ligament, and muscle (strain, sprain).
- Infections of the bone (osteomyelitis) or the joint (septic arthritis, transient synovitis) (see joint pain).
- Systemic disease like juvenile idiopathic arthritis, systemic lupus erythematosus (see joint pain with systemic disease).
- Orthopedic diseases like hip dislocation, Perthes disease, slipped capital femoral epiphysis (see above).
- Neurological conditions (spine, nerves) and tumors

Limping always needs to be taken seriously, and medical attention is necessary. See the doctor or go to the emergency room.

Usually, an x-ray is done, and an orthopedic surgeon is involved in the child's care.

Osteomyelitis. Osteomyelitis is an infection of the bone.

A bacterium called *Staphylococcus* is often the cause.

Symptoms are fever, pain, redness, warmth, swelling, and limited use of extremity.

Osteomyelitis can cause permanent bone damage.

Diagnosis is made by history, physical exam, x-ray, and bone scan if necessary.

Usually, an orthopedic surgeon is consulted.

Treatment: antibiotics for weeks and drainage if necessary.

Transient synovitis, septic arthritis (see joint pain).

Osteochondritis dissecant. Osteochondritis dissecant is a condition when bone and cartilage are separated from each other inside a joint, and a piece of bone can be loose there.

Symptoms are pain with movements and when the child puts weight on his leg. There is swelling and tenderness around the joint. The child might not be able to fully extend his arm or leg and feels that his joint is weak or "giving away."

The diagnosis is made by physical exam, x-ray, MRI, or CT scan. An orthopedic surgeon needs to see the child.

Treatment is rest and physical therapy. Surgery can be necessary.

Foreign bodies

One of the most important safety measures is not to give small objects like pennies, beans, corn, small Lego pieces, marbles, beads, buttons, thumbtacks, etc. to small children. Be sure that no parts of your child's toys can come off. Small batteries are particularly dangerous. It is also important not to give your baby or young child chunky foods, nuts, popcorn, grapes, cherry, and candy, or gum. Larger pieces of apple, carrot, celery, hot dog also can create problems because a small child can bite a piece off and choke. Meat that is not ground or cut to very tiny pieces also can cause choking. Do not let your young child run, walk, or play with food in his or her mouth.

If a child swallows a foreign body, it usually passes and can be found in the stool. But talk to the doctor. It is important to check every stool thoroughly to be sure it passed. If a battery is swallowed, the child needs to be taken to the emergency room right away.

A foreign body also can get stuck in the esophagus. In that case, the child gets frightened, grows pale, and cannot swallow. If the foreign object does not move, call 911. The foreign body needs to be removed. Also, when swallowing a foreign body, it can go the wrong way and end up in the airways.

If the airway is fully obstructed, the child chokes. He or she cannot speak, cough, or get air. The face turns purple, and the child loses consciousness. Different maneuvers are used depending on the child's age to expel the foreign body from the airways. They are taught in cardiorespiratory resuscitation (CPR) courses. You want to take that course.

If the child loses consciousness, CPR should be initiated, and a 911 call should be placed.

If the airway is partially blocked, the child will cough, and there will be some noise with the breathing (stridor) when he or she is breathing in. Often he or she seems to get better when the foreign body moves deeper in the airway. If the foreign body is not removed, infection can develop, like pneumonia. Foreign bodies in the bronchus can cause constant chronic cough and wheezing. If the child seems to have asthma but the medications to open up the airways (bronchodilators) do not work, foreign body can be the cause.

Children often put different things like rocks, beads, beans, corn, and whatnot into their mouth, ears, nose, genitals. When the foreign body is in the ear, the child usually complains of earache.

If the foreign body is in the nose for a while, the child has continuous nasal congestion, and a foul odor develops. If the foreign body is in the vagina, foul-smelling discharge will be the symptom.

Foreign bodies can injure the eye (see eye injuries).

Treatment: Many times if the foreign body is in the ear or nose, the doctor, often an ENT specialist, can pull out the object with a tweezer or with the help of a magnet or suction. However, sometimes surgery is necessary. In case of any foreign body, medical attention is needed. If the symptoms are severe, go to the emergency room, or call 911. Otherwise see the doctor as soon as possible.

Hair loss

The most common causes of hair loss:

- Young babies can have hair loss at the back of the head. They lie on their backs, and when moving their head, it rubs against the sheet. The hair grows back in a few months.
- Inflammation of the scalp, itchy skin on the scalp secondary to eczema, and seborrheic and atopic dermatitis can cause hair loss. Treatment with steroid ointment can help.
- *Ringworm-fungal infection* (*tinea capitis*). Small bumps develop on the scalp first, then a scaly, itchy reddish area appears. The infected hair is brittle, broken, and the consequence is hair loss.

  The area can get infected with bacteria, and small bumps with pus (pustula) can be seen. Boggy mass can also develop (*kerion*).

  Ultraviolet light (Wood's lamp) and microscopic exam of the hair can help to make the diagnosis.

  Treatment of the fungal infection is antifungal medication like Griseofulvin.
- Hair loss from *habitual hair pulling* (*trichotillomania*) is not very uncommon. Eyelashes and eyebrows can be affected as well.

  Treatment: Try to reduce anxiety. A psychologist might need to be involved in the child's care.

Headache

Important questions:

- When did the headache start?
- How often does the child have headaches?
- How long has the headache lasted?
- Is this the first time the child has had a headache?
- What time of the day has he or she experienced the headache?
- Does the headache wake him up?
- How bad was the headache?
- Where was it located?
- Is there a history of head injury?
- What kind of pain does the child get? Is it like pressure, or squeezing? Is it a sharp or dull pain, or is it a throbbing headache?
- Are there any other symptoms? Is there any vomiting or change of vision? Is the child sensitive to light? Is there any change of consciousness or behavior?
- What makes the headache better, and what makes it worse?
- Has the child taken any medicine for the pain? If the answer is yes, what medicine was taken, and did that help?
- Is there any vision change with the headache? Does the child see lights when he has the headache?
- Is there any other family member who gets headaches?
- Is there any family member who gets migraine headaches?

Acute headache. Headache can be the symptom of many acute illnesses. It can be a viral illness like influenza or bacterial illness like strep throat, sinusitis.

The child can take medicine for the pain, like acetaminophen or ibuprofen. The headache will disappear as the disease improves.

Headache, vomiting, fever. If the child has all of these symptoms, he or she needs to see the doctor soon. Lethargy is a condition when the child is sleepy and does not respond as usual. (If you talk to your child, he opens his eyes but falls back to sleep in a few seconds or a minute.) If lethargy, headache, fever, and vomiting are present, a more serious disease like meningitis is suspected. Urgent medical attention is needed. Go to the emergency room or call 911.

Headache and head injury. Headache is common after head injury. However, if there is a throbbing headache and change in consciousness, urgent medical attention is needed. Go to the emergency room or call 911. But if the child is unconscious, call 911. If the head injury is serious, neck injury is possible too. Therefore, do not move the child, keep him or her lying on the ground, keep the head still, and call 911.

Throbbing headaches and headaches that wake the child up at night always should be taken seriously and need to be investigated. See the doctor, but if the throbbing headache is severe, go to the emergency room.

After concussion, headaches are common and often last for a long time (see concussion).

Chronic headache. Headaches can last for a long time and frequently recur. Chronic headache can be caused by many ailments, like eye problems, high blood pressure, concussion, migraine, and stress. Many diseases also can be the cause of chronic headaches. Therefore, chronic headaches always need medical attention to try to find the possible underlying disease. However, if the headache wakes the child up at night, and/or projectile vomitings (the food comes up with force) accompanies the headache, an urgent doctor visit or emergency room visit is necessary. It can be a sign of increased pressure inside the head (increased intracranial pressure) that can affect the brain and can be a sign of tumor.

Migraine headaches. These are not uncommon in children. The pain is usually present on the side of the head but can be located in other places as well. Some children see light, and vomiting is not unusual. Migraine often starts with a so-called aura. Aura means some signs showing that migraine is coming. The child might see lights, has change of vision, may hear some singing, or may feel different. The child with migraine usually prefers to go to a dark room and sleep. Often others in the family have migraine headaches as well.

The child can take ibuprofen or Tylenol for the headache, but preventive medication can be necessary too. If a child has chronic headaches, a neurologist is often consulted.

Head—large, small, and misshapen

Large head (macrocephaly). If the baby's head size is over 97 percentile on the growth chart, he or she has a large head. In that case, close observation is necessary. So the circumference of the head is measured monthly.

It is important to know if the baby has any relatives with a large head.

If the growth of the head size is not abnormal, the baby develops normally, and if there is a relative with a large head, there is no worry.

But if the growth of the head size is too much and too fast, the soft spot is large, and the sutures are open, then further investigation is necessary. In this case, there is a suspicion that too much fluid is present in the chambers (ventricles) of the brain. This condition is called *hydrocephalus.*

Usually a head sonogram is done to make the diagnosis, but after the soft spot is closed, CT scan is necessary.

If the baby has this condition, a pediatric neurologist and a pediatric neurosurgeon will be consulted.

Small head (microcephaly). If the head circumference of a baby is less than 3 percentile on the growth chart, he or she has a small head. Close follow-up is needed. The head circumference is measured monthly. Let the doctor know if any of your relatives have a small head. If the head is constantly and normally growing and the baby's development is normal, then there is no problem. However, if the head does not grow or only very slowly and the baby is not developing or only developing very slowly, he or she can have a condition called microcephaly. In that case, there is a severe developmental problem and mental deficiency. Lately, Zika virus is found to be an agent causing microcephaly. (See infections that can harm the fetus.)

Misshapen head (plagiocephaly). The back of the head of babies is often flat. Since young infants stay on their back and do not move their head much, the pressure of the mattress is always at the same place, and that can result in flatness.

Placing the baby often on the stomach while you are there can help. Also if you approach the baby from both sides, it will make him or her move the head toward you.

This condition often resolves by itself.

However, if it is more significant and the head has some asymmetry, the condition is called *plagiocephaly*. The baby needs to see a craniofacial specialist who can give a helmet to correct the problem.

But there is a more significant condition when the head of the baby is misshapen. In that case, the soft spot and the sutures close early. That creates a problem because the brain does not have enough room to grow. This condition is called *craniosynostosis*. Some children have other abnormalities as well, like facial deformities. In this case, the multiple problems are called a syndrome. (Crouzon and Apert syndrome are such).

The baby will see a craniofacial specialist. Treatment is surgery.

Hearing and speech problems

For the normal development of speech and language, good hearing is essential. Therefore, the early detection of any hearing loss is very important.

The first screening test is due in the newborn nursery before the baby goes home. If the baby does not pass that test, it does not mean that he or she has hearing loss, but the test needs to be repeated. If the second test fails too, the baby needs to see an otolaryngologist (ear, nose, throat or ENT) specialist.

Signs that raise suspicion of hearing loss are the following:

- The baby does not respond to noises.
- The baby does not start to coo and squeal by six months of age.
- The baby does not start to babble by nine months of age.
- The baby does not say "ma-ma-ma, da-da-da" and does not imitate speech sounds by twelve months of age.
- No words like "mama" and "dada" by fifteen months of age.

Most hearing tests check on the child's response when hearing a sound.

One test that does not need the child's response is called auditory brainstem evoked response (ABER). That test checks the response of brain waves to sounds.

There are two types of hearing loss: conductive and sensorineural.

In *conductive hearing loss*, the sound cannot reach the inner ear because something blocks the way.

Causes:

- Frequent or not resolving ear infections (otitis media) that leads to accumulation of fluid in the middle ear
- Impacted wax
- Foreign body

In *sensorineural hearing loss*, the problem is at the inner ear, nerve (acoustic nerve), or brain.

It can be caused by the following:

- Structural defect.
- Maternal infection during pregnancy. Rubella is an example.
- Lack of oxygen (asphyxia).
- Severe jaundice.
- Disease of the central nervous system, like meningitis.
- Problem with mental development.
- Maternal alcohol abuse and fetal alcohol syndrome (see agents that can hurt the fetus).

If there is any suspicion of hearing loss, an otolaryngologist (ENT) should be consulted. An audiologist is also usually involved in the child's care.

Treatment depends on the cause.

If the child has conductive hearing loss, that is usually correctable.

If there is a chronic ear infection, ear tubes can help.

If there is impacted wax or foreign body, that needs to be removed.

If the child has sensorineural hearing loss, a consultation with an otologist specialist might be necessary. Constant loud noise also can cause hearing loss. Therefore, it is important to teach your child early on not to listen to very loud music, TV, radio, computer, etc. If your child plays a musical instrument, particularly drum, and plays loud music, have him use earplugs or ear muff.

For permanent hearing loss, the treatment can include hearing aids, speech therapy, and learning sign language. In some cases of sensorineural hearing loss, an implant placed to the inner ear (*cochlear implant*) could help.

Speech problems.

These can develop secondary to disorders that affect the coordination of muscles, as in cerebral palsy.

Developmental disorders can cause speech problems as well.

Articulation disorders. The child has a problem producing clear sounds, as in cerebral palsy.

Fluency disorder- stuttering. The child struggles to produce some words fluently, so tries it again and again.

Voice disorders. Hoarseness, stridor. Stridor is a hoarse sound with inspiration.

Newborns can have stridor secondary to structural problems in the larynx or trachea or softness of the cartilages. It often resolves by itself. But if the stridor is permanent and significant, an investigation is necessary by an ear, nose, and throat (ENT) doctor.

Hoarseness can be temporary from an illness, like laryngitis. Much shouting can cause chronic hoarseness from small nodes developing on the vocal cord. An ENT doctor is usually consulted.

Resonance disorders. The voice sounds like it comes from the nose. Enlarged adenoids and a problem with the soft palate like cleft palate can cause it.

Another cause of speech problems is autism (see behavioral problems).

Every child with a speech problem needs hearing and speech evaluation and speech therapy.

Heart problems, congestive heart failure

There are heart diseases which a child is born with (congenital heart diseases), and there are those that they get later in life (acquired heart diseases).

Congenital heart diseases

Some congenital heart diseases are diagnosed before the baby is born, with sonograms done during pregnancy.

Others are diagnosed in the nursery or in the first few days or weeks.

Before babies are discharged from the nursery, a screening test is done to look for heart diseases that did not show up during the nursery stay. The test is the checking of the baby's oxygenation. (See after birth.)

If a baby has poor appetite and poor weight gain and is irritable and sweating (at normal room temperature and without fever), has fast and hard breathing when fed, and/or the lips or face have a bluish color, congenital heart disease can be suspected. These symptoms also mean that the heart does not function normally and does not pump a sufficient amount of blood to the body (congestive heart failure).

Chest x-ray (CXR), electrocardiogram (ECG), echocardiogram (echo) help to make the diagnosis.

In some congenital heart diseases, the baby usually has good color (*acyanotic heart diseases*), like in ventricular septal defect (VSD), atrial septal defect (ASD), patent ductus arteriosus (PDA), or coarctation of the aorta.

Patent ductus arteriosus (PDA). Ductus arteriosus provides a communication between two main arteries of the body, the aorta and the pulmonary artery. It is open until birth, then it closes. But some babies have open ductus arteriosus even after birth, and that is a heart disease called patent ductus arteriosus (PDA).

Coarctation of aorta. This is a narrowing of the body's main artery (aorta). This condition leads to high blood pressure (hypertension).

Ventricular septal defect (VSD). In ventricular septal defect (VSD), there is a hole between the lower heart chambers (ventricles).

Atrial septal defect (ASD). In atrial septal defect (ASD), there is a hole between the upper heart chambers (atrium).

Some of these diseases can resolve spontaneously, but others may need surgery, depending on the severity.

There are some congenital heart diseases called *cyanotic heart diseases*, such as Tetralogy of Fallot and transposition of the great arteries. These are structural problems in the heart. The baby's lips, face, and fingernails are blue.

These heart diseases are usually severe and require surgery.

In tetralogy, the child can have so-called tetralogy spells. Suddenly the child gets irritable, the breathing is fast, and the bluish color increases. Placing the child in a knee-chest position can help, and call 911.

Acquired heart diseases

Endocarditis. Endocarditis is the infection and inflammation of the inner layer of the heart tissue including the heart valves. It occurs when germs spread through the bloodstream and attach to damaged areas of the heart. The damage can be caused by congenital heart disease or rheumatic fever.

Symptoms: fever, malaise, poor appetite, cough, weight loss. Fast heart beats and breathing can be present as well. ECG and echocardiogram (echo) help to make the diagnosis.

Treatment: rest and antibiotics.

Rheumatic fever is caused mostly by a bacteria called group A beta hemolytic streptococcus.

It can develop from a strep throat not treated or not sufficiently treated with antibiotics. Therefore, it is so important to see a doctor with a sore throat (see sore throat). The bacteria causes infection and inflammation of the heart valves.

If a child has had rheumatic fever and heart disease, he or she needs to take antibiotics regularly for years to prevent further heart damage.

Treatment of endocarditis is intravenous (into the vein) antibiotics.

Viruses, particularly Coxsackie B, can cause disease of the heart muscle (myocarditis).

Kawasaki disease can cause heart problems. The characteristic complication is a bulging and dilated area on the coronary artery (aneurysm). (See fever.)

Hypertrophic cardiomyopathy. Hypertrophic cardiomyopathy is the disease of the heart muscle. The heart gets enlarged.

The disease is inherited most of the time. It can start slowly, but it can progress fast. The child becomes exhausted with exercise.

If somebody has had this disease in your family, it is very important that you tell it to your child's doctor, because if the child has the disease, playing sports can be very dangerous. Before playing sports, the child needs to have a sports physical, including ECG and an echocardiogram (echo), a sonogram of the heart. He probably needs to see a cardiologist as well.

Myocarditis. Myocarditis is an inflammation of the heart muscle. Viral infections are often the cause of myocarditis. But there are other causes as well, like germs, toxins, and certain medications.

Symptoms are fever, rapid and difficult breathing, and rapid and abnormal heart rhythms (arrhythmias).

The diagnosis is made by chest x-ray, electrocardiogram (ECG), echocardiogram (echo) or cardiac MRI.

Treatment: rest and medications.

Usually a heart doctor (cardiologist) participates in the child's care.

Pericarditis. Pericardium is a sac that surrounds the heart.

Pericarditis is the inflammation of that sac (pericardium). It can be caused by a bacterial infection or a systemic disease, like rheumatic fever.

Symptoms are weakness, fever, chest pain, and shortness of breath.

Diagnosis is made by ECG, echo, and sometimes CT scan or MRI.

Treatment depends on the cause. If there is fluid accumulation in the sac, that needs to be drained surgically by a thoracic surgeon.

Heart rate

Children normally can have fast and slow heart rate, depending on what they are doing.

However, if the heart rate is extremely fast, like in supraventricular tachycardia (SVT), or extremely slow like in case of a heart block, serious problems can develop.

In case of *supraventricular tachycardia* (*SVT*), the child has a very fast heartbeat, color change, chest pain, and fast breathing. If the child has a conductive abnormality of the heart or *heart block* (*AV block*), the symptoms are very slow heartbeat, dizziness, being light-headed, and fainting. The diagnostic tool is ECG.

With any of these symptoms, the child needs to see the doctor, but with color change (extremely pale or bluish discoloration), difficulty breathing, fainting, urgent medical attention is necessary. Call 911. A cardiologist usually participates in the care of the child.

Treatment: medications and a pacemaker. This is a small device that is placed under the skin in the chest to help control heartbeats.

As I mentioned before, if the heart does not pump enough blood to the body, *congestive heart failure* (*CHF*) develops.

Infants with congestive heart failure have a poor appetite, are fussy, and have fast heartbeats and breathing, and sometimes color change.

If a child has congestive heart failure, the symptoms are fatigue, poor appetite, cough, fast heartbeat, difficulty breathing, and maybe color change. If there is difficulty breathing and bluish color, call 911.

A cardiologist is involved in the care of the child.

Treatment: oxygen and medications.

Some children with congenital or acquired heart disease need to take antibiotics before some surgeries and dental procedures to prevent further heart damage by a bacteria. The bacteria can cause infection and inflammation of the valves of the heart (endocarditis).

Rheumatic fever can cause endocarditis and permanent heart damage (see joint pain with systemic disease).

Heat- and cold-related illnesses

Heat exhaustion. Heat exhaustion is the consequence of profuse sweating that leads to dehydration.

Symptoms are the same as in dehydration: weakness, dizziness, pale skin, dry tongue, acetone smell in the breath, sunken eyes, and decreased urine output.

Treatment is replacement of the lost fluid and salt. If there is no vomiting, it can be done by drinking large amounts of fluids like Pedialyte for babies and younger children, or Gatorade for the older ones.

Urgent medical attention is needed. If the baby or child is lethargic or has no urine for eight to nine hours, go to the emergency room, or call 911.

Heat stroke. Heat stroke can develop with strenuous activities in hot and humid weather, when sweating is limited. Football players with heavy padding are at risk under those conditions. Young babies are sensitive to heat.

Symptoms are high fever, headache, nausea, dizziness. The skin is flushed, hot, and dry.

Loss of consciousness or seizure can develop.

Treatment is to remove the child's clothes, and place him or her in cold water. Do not bring the temperature down below 102 degrees Fahrenheit or 39 degrees Celsius.

Urgent medical attention is necessary. Go to the emergency room, but if there is loss of consciousness or seizure activity, call 911.

However, the best treatment is prevention. Do not let your child stay out in the heat very long. Do not let him or her exercise for a long time in hot weather.

Use sunscreen to avoid sunburn.

Never leave your child in the car alone.

Cold injury, frostbite, and hypothermia. Frostbite causes injury of the tissues secondary to freezing.

Frostbites are graded by their severity, like burns.

In first-degree frostbites, the skin is red, maybe with some swelling.

In second-degree frostbites, blisters are present.

In third-degree frostbites, there is necrosis.

Symptoms are itching, numbness, prickly sensation, burning, and tenderness. The pain and tenderness can last for a long time. The skin is red or white.

Bacterial infection can develop.

Treatment is proper warming. The water should be only slightly warmer than the body temperature. Do not rub the frozen area with snow or ice, and do not use direct heat, but it is good to move the affected area. Medical attention is necessary.

Prevention is important.

Avoid exposure of your child's face to cold weather and direct contact with cold objects, because exposure to cold can cause direct trauma and rash.

Limit the time your child spends outdoors in cold, wet, and windy weather.

Have your child dress in several layers of warm clothing.

Have him wear a hat that fully covers the ears, mittens, and warm socks and shoes.

Hypothermia. If the child's body is exposed to extremely cold weather, so-called hypothermia can develop.

The body temperature falls to 95 degrees Fahrenheit or 35 degrees Celsius. This is a dangerous situation.

Symptoms are shivering, clumsiness, drowsiness, and muscle weakness. Loss of consciousness can develop.

Move the child to the closest warm place. If the cloth is wet, change it to dry warm cloth. Put a blanket around him. In the meantime, 911 should be called.

Hepatitis

The most common causes of hepatitis are viruses.

Viral hepatitis causes the inflammation of the liver. It is contagious.

Symptoms are jaundice, the yellow discoloration of the skin and the white part of the eye (sclera) (see jaundice), poor appetite, tiredness, nausea or vomiting, abdominal pain, enlarged liver. The urine is dark, and the stool has a light color.

In case of hepatitis B, rash and joint pain can occur too.

Often a child with hepatitis has no jaundice or may not have any symptoms.

If a child has jaundice, the bilirubin test (blood test) shows that the direct bilirubin is elevated (see jaundice).

If a blood test shows elevated liver enzymes, hepatitis is a possibility.

The presence of hepatitis antigens confirms the diagnosis.

Hepatitis A. Hepatitis A infections spread with contaminated food, water, and from infected persons.

The incubation period for hepatitis A is 15 to 50 days.

Prevention: Hepatitis A vaccine is included in the immunization schedule.

If a child is exposed to hepatitis A, immunoglobulin is given.

Hepatitis B and C. These are transmitted by blood, secretions, open wounds, and sexual contact.

The incubation period for hepatitis B is 45 to 160 days.

There are also hepatitis B carriers, who do not have symptoms but carry and transmit the disease.

Hepatitis B and C also can be transmitted from the mother to the newborn baby.

To prevent the development of hepatitis B, the baby receives Hepatitis B immunoglobulin (HBIG) within hours after birth. He or she also gets the first hepatitis B vaccine at the same time to start to develop immunity against the disease.

After the baby of a Hepatitis B–infected mother has received the three hepatitis B vaccines, blood test is needed to check for antigens and antibody levels. If the antibody level is low, a fourth shot is necessary. If a child is in close contact with someone who has hepatitis B, HBIG is needed for prevention as well.

Hepatitis B shot is included in the immunization schedule.

For hepatitis C, recently a cure has been developed. A medication called Harvoni is taken by mouth.

Hepatitis D. This infection only affects persons who have hepatitis B.

Hepatitis E. This is transmitted by contaminated water or by blood. Symptoms are the same as with other forms of hepatitis.

A vaccine exists but is not used in the USA.
Hepatitis can lead to liver failure.

Other agents and conditions that can cause hepatitis:

- Epstein BARR (EB) virus that causes mononucleosis, and cytomegalovirus that can cause severe congenital infections and similar symptoms like mononucleosis.
- Autoimmune diseases like lupus. (See joint pain with systemic diseases.)
- Poisons and medications.
- Problems with the tubes that transport bile from the liver (bile ducts). These ducts can be narrow or blocked (*biliary atresia*). The disease is severe but fortunately rare.
- *Choledochal cyst* is a bulging (dilatation) of the bile ducts. The main symptom in both conditions is jaundice that does not resolve during the first two months of life. Blood test shows that the direct bilirubin is elevated. (See jaundice.) Treatment is surgery.

Hernias

There are different types of hernias.

Inguinal hernia. This is the most common hernia in children. The inguinal hernia appears close to the groin area—in boys at the scrotum, and in girls at the labia. There is swelling there that is caused by a protruding part of the intestine getting through a weak area of the abdominal wall.

Femoral hernia. This appears at the inner thigh.

These hernias can be *strangulated* (*incarcerated*) *hernia.* The symptoms are severe abdominal pain, vomiting, and a swollen abdomen. The lump is tender and the hernia cannot be reduced (placed back).
If your child has these symptoms, go to the emergency room, or call 911 right away.
Treatment is surgery.

Umbilical hernia. This is not uncommon in young babies. The belly button is enlarged and bulging.
Umbilical hernia usually does not cause problems and often spontaneously resolves.

Hiatal hernia. In case of hiatal hernia, the upper part of the stomach protrudes into the chest cavity through an opening of the diaphragm that separates the abdominal and chest cavity.
Symptoms of gastroesophageal reflux disease (GERD) are present.
Surgery is rarely necessary. (See vomiting.)

Hoarseness

If your child is hoarse, his voice is raspy and deeper than usual.

Hoarseness is usually caused by viral infections, like the "common cold."

Laryngitis, gastroesophageal reflux, and overuse of the vocal cord with frequent shouting, loud singing, etc. can cause hoarseness.

If your child is hoarse and it does not improve in a couple of days, see the doctor.

But if the child has a raspy sound when breathing in, like having croup, go to see the doctor at once. However, if there is trouble breathing as well, go to the emergency room, or call 911.

Infectious diseases of childhood

Most of these infectious diseases are more common in childhood than later on. The reason for this is that by adulthood, most people develop immunity against these diseases. Either they were exposed to the disease or they received protective shots, immunizations (see immunizations).

These diseases, with the exception of scarlet fever, whooping cough, and diphtheria, result in lifetime immunity.

So if someone had the disease as a child, he will not get it as an adult. However, if a child had chickenpox, he can have shingles as an adult. Most of these diseases are not common anymore, thanks to vaccinations.

These diseases are contagious, and most of them are caused by viruses. The exceptions are diphtheria, scarlet fever, and whooping cough.

This chapter will make you familiar with the symptoms of these infectious diseases, so if your child exhibits some of these symptoms, keep him or her at home, and contact the doctor.

Chickenpox. Chickenpox is very contagious, caused by the varicella-zoster virus. Incubation period is about fourteen days.

At the beginning of the disease, red spots, bumps, then blisters appear. The blisters can be located anywhere on the skin and scalp. They are itchy, and the child is scratching. Blisters also can develop in the mouth.

Fever is common.

New blisters can develop for the next few days. The blisters gradually change to scabs.

All stages of the rash can be present at the same time as bumps, blisters, and scabs.

Usually, after one week the child has only scabs. At that time, he or she is not contagious anymore and can return to school.

Chickenpox can have complications.

Scratching of the blisters can lead to local infections. Redness, warmth, tenderness, and swelling of the area are the symptoms. If your child exhibits these symptoms, call the doctor.

Chickenpox can affect the central nervous system (encephalitis). So if the child has vomiting, headache, change of consciousness, go to the emergency room, or call 911.

Pneumonia also can develop. If the child has high fever and coughing, call the doctor. However, if your child has trouble breathing, go to the emergency room or call 911.

Do not give aspirin when your child has chickenpox because severe disease *Reye's syndrome* can develop. Liver and brain damage can be the consequence. Symptoms are vomiting, headache, lethargy (the child always falls back to sleep even when you talk to him or her). Seizures can develop as well.

Chickenpox gives lifetime immunity.

Chickenpox is dangerous to pregnant women because it can severely affect the fetus (see agents that can harm the fetus).

As I mentioned before, one can develop *shingles* many years later following chickenpox infection.

Vaccine is available to prevent chickenpox (Varivax).

Children whose fighting capability against infections is weak (immunocompromised), and young babies exposed, can receive varicella-zoster immune globulin (VZIG) for protection.

There is also a vaccine for adults to prevent shingles.

Measles. Measles is a contagious disease caused by a virus. Incubation period is ten to twelve days, then the cold symptoms start, and on the fourteenth day, the rash appears.

Since it starts like a cold, the history of exposure is very important.

Symptoms are runny nose, sneezing, coughing, watery pink eyes, fever, and malaise.

When the rash appears, red spots on the face, behind the ears, and all over the body can be seen.

Two days later, the temperature drops, and the child feels better.

After the rash is gone, the disease is over.

Complications most commonly are ear infection and pneumonia. But the disease can affect the nervous system as well (encephalitis). If there is vomiting, headache, and lethargy, go to the emergency room, or call 911.

Immunity is lifelong.

- Vaccine is available to prevent measles: MMR (measles, mumps, rubella).

Immune globulin can help to prevent the disease of an exposed baby or an immunocompromised child.

Rubella (German measles). Rubella is a contagious disease caused by a virus.

The incubation period is two to three weeks.

Symptoms are fever, pink eye, rash. The rash consists of small pink spots. They can be seen on the face, behind the ears, and all over the body.

There are also enlarged lymph nodes, most often at the back of the head (occiput).

After the rash is gone in three to four days, the disease is over.

Immunity is lifelong.

Rubella is dangerous to pregnant women because it can severely affect the fetus (see agents that can harm the fetus).

Protective shot is available: MMR (measles, mumps, rubella).

Mumps. Mumps is a contagious disease caused by a virus. The incubation period is two to three weeks.

The characteristic symptom is the swelling of the parotid gland that is located in front of the ear. The swelling can be on one or both sides. Other salivary glands can be swollen too, like the ones under the chin.

Chewing is often painful, and earache is a frequent complaint. One can have mumps without the swelling of the gland, only having fever.

But swelling of the parotid gland can also develop from bacterial infection or viral infection other than mumps.

The disease lasts for about a week, and when the swelling is gone, the disease is over.

Mumps can have complications. It can affect the nervous system. Symptoms are severe vomiting, fever, headache, lethargy (meningoencephalitis). Mumps also can cause severe abdominal pain and vomiting from the inflammation of the pancreas (pancreatitis). If these symptoms are present, go to the emergency room, or call 911.

If a child gets mumps after puberty, in boys, swelling of the testicles with pain can develop. Girls can have abdominal pain caused by the inflammation of an ovary.

Lifelong immunity develops after mumps.

Vaccine is available to prevent mumps (MMR [measles, mumps, and rubella]).

Roseola. Roseola is a contagious disease caused by a virus, generally in the first two years. The incubation period is about ten days.

The disease starts with high fever that lasts for three days without any other symptoms.

The child does not feel or look bad even with high fever.

After three days, the fever breaks, and a rash develops. These are pink spots on the face, behind the ears, and all over the body. The diagnosis of roseola only can be made when the rash appeared. Until then, there can only be a suspicion.

After a few days, the rash goes away, and the disease is over.

Complication of roseola can be seizure from the high fever. Therefore, it is important to give the child fever reducer.

Fifth disease. Fifth disease is a contagious disease caused by the virus parvovirus B19. It is not as highly contagious as the other diseases described above.

The incubation period is four to fourteen days but can be as long as twenty-one days.

It usually starts with redness of the face, so-called slapped face, then a pink rash appears. The rash is more prominent on the extremities, mostly on the arms and thighs, but can be present on the trunk as well. The rash has a lacelike appearance. Even after the rash seems to fade out, it often reappears after sun exposure, sweating, or a warm bath.

The rash can last for weeks, but the child does not feel bad. Complications are rare.

After the rash develops, the child can go to school because at that point, he or she is not considered to be contagious anymore.

Scarlet fever (scarlatina). Scarlet fever is a contagious disease caused by a germ called *group A Streptococcus.* This germ most commonly causes sore throat and tonsillitis (strep throat) but also often causes skin and other infections.

The incubation period is three to five days.

Scarlet fever used to be a feared disease decades ago, but with the discovery of penicillin, now it is treated as a strep throat. Symptoms are fever, sore throat, vomiting, sometimes abdominal pain. A very faint-red rash appears, mostly on the abdomen, chest, and inner part of the arms. The rash is rough to touch. The rash is characteristic of scarlet fever but is not always present. However, a red throat and changed appearance of the tongue can be seen. The tongue can be red with red bumps (strawberry tongue) or coated, white with red bumps (white strawberry tongue). After the rash is gone, the disease is over.

Treatment of scarlet fever and strep throat is extremely important. If it is not treated or not sufficiently treated, acute rheumatic fever can develop that can lead to heart disease (see heart problems). Also, a kidney disease (acute glomerulonephritis) can be the consequence of an infection with group A Streptococcus (see bloody urine).

The treatment is an antibiotic, usually penicillin, often amoxicillin. Be sure that your child takes it precisely and finishes the whole course, ten days, even if she feels better after a few days.

Whooping cough (pertussis). Whooping cough is a contagious disease caused by a germ called *Bordetella pertussis.*

The incubation period is one to two weeks, and the disease can last for a couple of months.

The younger the child is, the more severe the disease is.

Symptoms are like that of a cold (upper respiratory infection) in the beginning, with cough, runny nose, and slight fever. That lasts for about two weeks.

After that the cough gets severe. The child gets coughing spells and can have problems getting air. After the coughing spell, often there is a loud inspiration with a whoop. Babies get a severe cough but without the whoop. Also, they can stop breathing (apnea). Because of the troubled breathing, young babies are often hospitalized.

Vomiting is frequent after the cough.

The last two to three weeks of the disease is recovery, when the cough gradually disappears.

The most common complication of whooping cough is pneumonia. Dehydration also can be a problem from vomiting, and since eating can trigger coughing spells, the child is afraid to eat or drink.

Therapy is erythromycin or azithromycin. The same drugs are used for prophylaxis of an exposed child.

Pertussis shots are available. Pertussis shot is included in the DTaP (diphtheria, tetanus, pertussis), Pentacel (diphtheria, tetanus, pertussis, polio, HIB), and VAXELIS (diphtheria, tetanus, pertussis, polio, hepatitis B, HIB) vaccines to prevent whooping cough.

The immunity fades with time. Adults can have whooping cough, but they usually have a mild disease.

However, they can transfer the disease to babies. Therefore, it is recommended for mothers and caretakers to get the Tdap shot if they have not had it in the past ten years. That way they can protect the baby they care for.

Pregnant women are recommended to receive Tdap prenatally, but if it was not given then, they should have it after delivery. The antibodies the baby gets from the mother help to protect him or her in the first few months.

Diphtheria. Diphtheria is a contagious disease caused by a germ called *Corynebacterium diphtheriae.* The incubation period is two to seven days.

Thanks to immunizations, this disease is rare.

Symptoms are fever and sore throat. Then a membrane is formed on the throat. If it spreads to the voice box (larynx), a barking cough, hoarseness, and difficulty breathing develops. The child can choke as well if the membrane blocks the airway. The heart (myocarditis) and the nerves (neuritis) can be affected too.

Therapy is antibiotics and antitoxin.

After the disease, the child needs immunization against diphtheria with DTaP or Tdap shot because the disease does not give lifelong immunity.

Prevention is diphtheria, tetanus and pertussis (DTaP or Tdap) vaccine.

Hepatitis. Hepatitis is a disease of the liver and most often caused by viruses. The most common forms are hepatitis A, B, C, D, and E (see hepatitis).

Itchy skin

Different conditions can cause itching, and usually a rash is present as well.

Common causes of itching:

- Dry skin
- Seborrheic dermatitis
- Allergic rash—hives (see allergies)
- Eczema—atopic dermatitis
- Poison ivy
- Psoriasis
- Diaper rash, particularly if it is caused by a yeast infection (monilial dermatitis)
- Skin parasite (scabies)
- Rectal itching can be caused by pinworms

Treatment for dry skin is simply a good moisturizer (Aveeno, Eucerin, Aquaphor, Cetaphil, Dove, etc.).

Some infants have *cradle cap* (*seborrhea capitis*). That is the crusting and scaling of some areas or the whole scalp. It can be removed with a cotton ball soaked in baby oil. You squeeze the oil out, and gently rub the scalp with the cotton ball. If the cradle cap is thick, you can put baby oil on the scalp at night, and wash it off the next morning.

Seborrheic dermatitis. The skin is red and scaly.
Treatment: local use of steroids can be helpful.

Monilial diaper rash. Monilial diaper rash is caused by a yeast called *monilia.* The skin is red with small bumps.
Treatment is antifungal cream, like nystatin.

This diaper rash is often accompanied with white spots in the mouth, another manifestation of a yeast infection (oral thrush). That is treated with antifungal nystatin drops. If the diaper rash gets worse, or does not improve after you treated it for a week, see the doctor.

Ringworm. Ringworm is a skin infection caused by a fungus (tinea). It is a red itchy rash that looks like a ring with prominent border. It can appear anywhere on the skin.

Treatment is antifungal medicine.

Scabies. Scabies is caused by a skin parasite. It is contagious and easily transmitted by skin-to-skin contact. If a child has a very itchy rash with small skin-colored bumps, he or she probably has scabies. Often a family member or a friend has it as well.

The location is often the hand, in between the fingers, wrist, ankle, genital area but can be present anywhere on the skin.

The skin can get infected from the constant scratching.

Treatment is permethrin cream (Elimite). It is applied to the whole body from the chin down at bedtime and washed off the next morning. Babies can have scabies on their face, and in that case, the face should be treated as well. After that, the child is not contagious and can attend school. Usually one treatment is sufficient. If the itching continues, maybe another treatment is needed in two weeks. The bedding and cloth needs to be washed. Everybody in the same household should be treated at the same time as well.

Poison ivy. If a child has blisters on the skin with oozing and crusting, particularly if some of the blisters are linear, poison ivy is most likely responsible for the development of the rash.

Usually there is also a history that the child was in the woods.

It is a dermatitis with intense itching that can be caused by other plants, like poison oak and poison sumac as well. Treatment: steroid ointment, and if the dermatitis is more severe, steroid by mouth.

If your child is suspected of having poison ivy, see the doctor.

Atopic dermatitis—eczema (see allergies)

Psoriasis. Psoriasis is a chronic skin condition that can occur at any age.

If a child has psoriasis, there are pink areas and dry scaly patches on the skin. The dry skin can crack, and the sores can bleed. The skin is itchy.

Treatment consists of topical ointments, creams, ultraviolet lights, and sometimes medications.

Jaundice

Jaundice is the yellow discoloration of the skin and the white area of the eyes (sclera).

The yellow color of the eyes is important, because if a baby eats too much yellow vegetables, like carrots or sweet potatoes, the skin gets yellow, but the eyes do not.

So in this case, the baby does not have jaundice. What he or she has is called *hypercarotenemia*. On the other hand, a baby or a child can have jaundice without the skin turning yellow, but the color of the eyes shows that he or she has jaundice.

During the first few days of life, newborns often have jaundice. It is normal most of the time, and the condition is called *physiologic jaundice*. Breastfed babies can develop jaundice in the first week of life, called *breastfeeding jaundice*. It usually develops on the second or third day. The degree of jaundice is measured by the level of bilirubin in the blood. It can be checked by a blood test or through the skin (transcutaneous bilirubin test). The two measurements can differ, but only a little. If the transcutaneous bilirubin level is high, the blood test should be checked. If the bilirubin level is elevated, the baby's doctor will decide if treatment is necessary or if only follow-up is required.

For a high bilirubin level, the treatment is usually phototherapy. The baby is placed under a special blue light that breaks down the bilirubin. The baby can lose fluid under the light because of sweating and more frequent loose stools. Therefore, proper fluid intake is important. The baby's eyes are covered for protection from the light. Be sure that the cover fits well and is always in place. You should not directly look at the light because that can hurt your eye.

Exchange blood transfusion is rarely needed. An exchange blood transfusion removes a certain amount of blood of the patient and replaces it with donor blood to remove abnormal blood components, in this case bilirubin.

High bilirubin levels are usually caused by so-called blood *incompatibility*. This means that the blood type of the mother and the blood type of the baby differ. If the mother's blood type is Rh negative and the baby has Rh positive blood, *Rh incompatibility* exists. Rh factor is an inherited protein on the surface of the red blood cells. If the baby has this protein, he is Rh-positive; if not, he is Rh-negative.

Also, if the mother has O positive blood and the baby has A or B blood type, *ABO incompatibility* exists. Rh-negative mothers need a RhoGAM shot after delivery to prevent high bilirubin levels of the next baby. Bilirubin levels are higher with subsequent pregnancies.

If the jaundice starts early, on the first day, and the bilirubin level is high or increases rapidly and a blood test called Coombs test is positive, treatment probably will be necessary. Coombs test is routinely checked on all babies after birth. Coombs test detects antibodies that can destroy the baby's red blood cells.

Premature babies are more sensitive to high bilirubin levels because their liver is less mature. Therefore, treatments are often initiated even if the bilirubin level is not that high.

In certain anemias, there is a *destruction of the red blood cells* after the newborn period, as in the case of sickle cell anemia, thalassemia or certain *enzyme defects* of the red blood cells (glucose-6-phosphate deficiency, or pyruvate kinase deficiency). As a consequence, jaundice develops in these diseases.

Infections also can cause increased bilirubin levels.

It is important to treat high bilirubin levels because it can cause brain damage (*kernicterus*).

If the jaundice lasts longer than four weeks, it is called *prolonged jaundice*, and the baby needs a checkup. It can be normal, but it also can be a sign of an underlying problem like a choledochal cyst. *Choledochal cyst* is a rare congenital anomaly. The common bile duct (tube) called ductus choledochus that transports bile from the liver to the gallbladder and small intestine has swelling (dilatation). Consequently, bile may back up in the liver. Therapy is surgery.

After the neonatal period is over, jaundice is always a very significant symptom that requires medical attention.

Bilirubin has two fractions: indirect and direct bilirubin. All of the conditions mentioned so far are associated with elevated indirect bilirubin level but the choledochal cyst. Increased direct bilirubin level reflects on the liver. So if that is elevated, liver disease like hepatitis (see hepatitis) or problem with the bile (biliary system) is suspected. Blockage in the tubes (obstruction of the ducts) transporting the bile inside the liver *biliary atresia* and choledochal cyst causes jaundice, liver damage, and liver failure. The direct bilirubin is elevated.

Congenital (hereditary) spherocytosis causes jaundice and anemia (see anemia).

Sickle cell disease and thalassemia are hemoglobin defects. They can cause jaundice as well (see anemia).

Jerking and strange movements

Jerking and seizures. Jerking of the whole body or part of the body is most often a manifestation of a seizure.

If the seizure stops by the time the doctor sees the child, the important questions you need to answer are the following:

- What happened?
- Did the child lose consciousness?
- Did the child fall? Did he or she sustain any injuries?
- Was the whole body, or parts of the body jerking? Which parts?
- Did the child have a fever? If yes, what was the temperature?
- Was there vomiting, diarrhea, or any other symptoms?
- Did the child take any drugs?
- Was the child sick before it happened?
- When did the jerking start, and how long did it last?
- Did he have foaming at the mouth?
- Did the child bite his tongue?
- Did the child wet his pants?
- Did the child fall asleep after the seizure?
- Has the child had any seizure activity in the past?
- Is there anybody in the family who ever had a seizure?

Jerking can occur without being a seizure, for example, when the child is sleeping or just waking up. But also, seizures can occur during sleep.

The most dramatic form of seizure is called *grand mal seizure.*

The child loses consciousness, and the whole body is jerking (convulsion). Foaming saliva comes out of the mouth, and the clenched teeth can cause tongue injury. The child can wet his or her pants, and vomiting can occur. The tongue can block the airways and cause choking. A series of seizures is called *status epilepticus.* The child does not regain consciousness between seizures. That is a true emergency. Call 911.

Some children have a seizure with fever, called *febrile seizure*. It is caused by rapidly increasing temperatures. Febrile seizures can recur, but benign febrile seizures have no consequences. After six years of age, febrile seizures stop.

It is very important that the doctor checks the child even if the seizure spontaneously stopped. The doctor must find out if any cause for the seizure can be identified. Fever and seizure can be caused by severe infections of the central nervous system, like meningitis.

If your child has a seizure for the first time, call 911. Also call if the seizure lasts longer than five minutes.

If the child has no fever and the episode recurs regularly, *epilepsy* is suspected. Electroencephalograph (EEG), which examines brain electric activity, can confirm the diagnosis. EEG is not necessary after a single febrile seizure. Anyway, the EEG is often normal after febrile seizures.

You want to be sure to prevent any harm that the seizure can cause.

Prevent injury from falling, remove furniture, and other objects close to the child. Place him or her on the side, and turn the head to the side. That prevents the aspiration of vomit and obstruction of the airway by the tongue. Do not try to hold the child down to try to stop the jerking, and do not put anything to his mouth. After the seizure, the child falls asleep (postictal state).

When seizures recur in case of epilepsy, the child often has discomfort, stomachache, and the feeling that a seizure is coming. This phenomenon is called aura.

Tetanus can cause severe, life-threatening seizures (see cuts and lacerations).

The treatment of acute grand mal seizure is a drug called diazepam. It can be given through a vein (intravenously) or per rectum (rectally). After the first seizure, it is good to keep rectal diazepam (Diastat) at home.

There are other types of seizures too, not as dramatic as grand mal seizure but still important. The child can just stare, not respond to questions, drop things, or fall. These are signs of *petit mal or absence seizures.* These seizures can happen quite a few times before it is recognized that the child has a seizure disorder.

Another type of seizure is when the child is either conscious or not, and only certain parts of the body are jerking. That is called *partial or focal seizure.*

Another type of seizure is called *myoclonic seizure,* when the child is conscious and only certain muscles jerk.

There is a type of seizure that usually starts around six months of age. The symptoms are fast, frequent recurring bowing of the head, bending of the trunk and the hip. The arms are extended. The name of this type of seizure is *infantile spasms.* Infantile spasm can cause developmental disabilities.

There are certain triggers provoking seizures, like light exposure or sleep deprivation.

For the treatment of epilepsy, there are different medications used, depending on the type of the seizure. The drug levels are monitored by blood tests to have the right amount of medicine in the blood. The normal blood level reassures that the dose of the medicine is appropriate to prevent seizures but does not cause side effects.

Be sure that the medicine is not stopped even when the child is doing well. Sudden withdrawal of medication can provoke seizure. A neurologist is usually involved in the child's care with epilepsy. He or she will check the EEG and taper off the medicine if the child is seizure-free for a certain amount of time, at least a couple of years.

It is important that the child does not participate in sports that would endanger him or her. Also be sure that the child has constant supervision when swimming or being in the water.

Strange movements

Tics. Tics are uncontrollable, rapid muscle movements.

The most common forms are blinking, jerking of the face, head, neck, shrugging of the shoulder, clearing the throat.

The child has more tics when anxious, but he or she can suppress them for a while. Simple tics usually disappear.

Treatment: There is no specific treatment, but it is best to ignore them and decrease stress as much as possible.

Tourette's syndrome. When the child has multiple tics and makes involuntary noises like sniffing, throat clearing, saying words without intention, often repeating them, and using obscene language, Tourette's syndrome is suspected.

In case of Tourette's syndrome, a neurology consult is needed.

Chorea (Sydenham's chorea). This illness is secondary to *group A Streptococcus* infection that is causing strep throat, tonsillitis, scarlet fever.

Symptoms of chorea are jerking movements and clumsiness. The muscle tone is decreased. There are extreme mood swings. Speech can be affected as well.

It usually disappears in weeks or months.

It can be prevented by the effective treatment of strep infections.

There is another disease called chorea (Huntington's chorea). Some of the symptoms are similar, but that is severe inherited neurologic disease.

Impaired coordination—acute ataxia. A child who has ataxia is clumsy. His or her movements are not well coordinated. The gait is wide based and unsteady. Involuntary shaking (tremor), decreased muscle tone, and abnormal eye movement can be present as well.

It can be caused by many conditions, most commonly by intoxication, trauma, infection, or any event in the central nervous system. It also can be hereditary.

Suddenly developed acute ataxia can be resolved spontaneously.

If the ataxia is constant and chronic, that suggests a serious problem.

If a child has ataxia, urgent medical attention is needed.

Usually a neurologist is consulted.

Joint pain

Joint pain should always be taken seriously. The same is true for limping, with or without joint pain.

The most common cause of joint pain is injury. In case of injury, history is important. Often injury of the skin can be seen (abrasion, laceration, or bruise).

The most common symptoms are swelling and pain of the extremity with movements. If the skin over the painful joint is also red and warm, infection is likely. It can be caused by viruses or bacteria.

After viral infection, the so-called *transient synovitis* can develop.

The child has pain, usually in one of the joints, most often in the hip or the knee. Limping is often present. This is a self-limited condition.

Bacterial infection is the cause of *septic arthritis*.

Most often the larger joints are involved, like the hip and knee.

Symptoms are swollen joint, pain, and restricted movements. The skin is red and warm above the joint. The child often has a fever. But sometimes the symptoms are not that obvious. The disease can start insidiously and still causes severe destruction of the joint.

Blood tests suggesting infection help to make the diagnosis.

If septic arthritis is suspected, fluid is removed from the joint for both diagnostic and therapeutic purposes. The fluid will be sent to the laboratory for analysis and for culture to find out what is the bacteria that caused the infection. The drainage of the fluid also will decrease the pain and improve movements.

Other diagnostic studies are x-ray, MRI, and bone scan. They are often necessary to make the diagnosis.

An orthopedic surgeon needs to be involved in the child's care.

Treatment: Intravenous (IV) antibiotic for weeks. Sometimes surgery is necessary.

Joint pain also can be caused by diseases that involve different organs in the body, like lupus erythematosus, juvenile rheumatoid arthritis, and Lyme disease. (See joint pain with systemic diseases.)

Osteochondritis dissecans. In case of osteochondritis dissecans, a piece of bone or cartilage breaks off and moves in the joint, and consequently, pain develops. Treatment is surgery (see flat foot and other orthopedic problems).

Perthes disease and slipped capital femoral epiphysis are also causes of joint pain. (See flatfoot and other orthopedic problems.)

Joint pain with systemic disease

Rheumatic fever. Rheumatic fever develops one to three weeks after a strep throat. The germ causing the strep throat is *group A beta hemolytic Streptococcus.*

Rheumatic fever has so-called major and minor manifestations. The major manifestations are the following:

- Heart disease (carditis).
- Inflammation of large joints, like hips, knees, ankles, shoulders, elbows, wrists (polyarthritis). The pain can move from joint to joint.
- Constant strange movements (chorea) (see jerking and strange movements).
- Rash consisting of faint pink circles (erythema marginatum).
- Small nodes under the skin, around the joints (subcutaneous nodules).

The minor manifestations are the following:

- Fever and malaise
- Joint pain (arthralgia)
- Electrocardiogram (ECG) changes
- Abnormal blood test results (elevated sedimentation rate-ESR, or C-reactive protein-CRP), including confirmation of a strep infection with a positive strep culture, showing the presence of the germ or elevated antistreptolysin O titer-ASO titer

Treatments:

- Steroids.
- Salicylates like aspirin.
- A course of penicillin, then daily penicillin for prophylaxis for years to prevent another strep infection. That is very

important because a new strep infection can damage the heart.

Since strep throat can cause severe secondary diseases, heart and kidney disease, and Sydenham chorea, it is most important to have a medical checkup if your child has any sore throat. In case of strep throat, complete a ten-day course of antibiotic therapy without skipping a dose.

Juvenile idiopathic arthritis (JIA). JIA is a chronic disease that can affect one or more joints.

The symptoms are swelling, often redness and warmth of the joint. Motion of the joint is limited secondary to pain.

The disease can also involve other organs of the body, like the eyes (uveitis), heart, liver and kidneys.

Systemic manifestations are fever, rash, decreased appetite, enlarged lymph nodes, liver, and spleen.

There is no specific test to diagnose juvenile rheumatoid arthritis, but there are tests to support the diagnosis: ESR, CRP, rheumatoid factor, antinuclear antibody test—ANA.

Treatment:

- Salicylates like aspirin
- Nonsteroidal anti-inflammatory drugs like naproxen and ibuprofen
- Steroids
- Immunosuppressive anticancer drugs
- Physiotherapy
  A rheumatologist is involved in the care of the child.

Lupus erythematosus or systemic lupus erythematosus (SLE). Lupus is a chronic disease affecting the connective tissues of the body, like ligaments and tendons.

It also can affect the blood vessels, the skin, and different organs.

The cause is unknown, but it seems that there is a problem with the body's immune system. The role of the immune system is to fight infections. The problem seems to be in lupus that the body cannot distinguish between foreign cells like germs and the body's own cells. Consequently, the body's own cells get destroyed as well.

The symptoms are fever, weakness, tiredness, and often joint pain and swelling. A rash can occur, and it is usually located on the nose, called butterfly rash. Sun exposure often makes the rash worse. Enlargement of the lymph nodes, liver, and spleen are common.

Other organs often involved are heart, lung, kidneys, bowels, eyes, and the nervous system.

Diagnosis is made by the clinical picture and a positive laboratory test, ANA.

However, the lab test alone is not enough to make the diagnosis. Treatment:

- Nonsteroidal anti-inflammatory drugs like naproxen
- Steroids
- Immunosuppressive, anticancer drugs

A rheumatologist is usually involved in the care of the child with lupus erythematosus (LE).

Lyme disease

Lyme disease is caused by a microorganism called spirochete. It is transmitted to people by a deer tick bite. It is hard to find the small sesame-seed-size tick.

Incubation period is three to thirty-two days but usually one to two weeks.

Symptoms:

The most important symptom to make the diagnosis is a circular red area that develops at the site of the tick bite. It gradually gets bigger and bigger (*erythema migrans*). However, this rash does not always develop if someone has Lyme disease.

Fever, malaise, headache, and muscle pain are often present in the early stage of the disease. Joint pain often develops, usually affecting the large joints, mostly the knees.

After weeks, in the late stage of the disease, it can affect different organs. Joins can be swollen, painful with restricted movements, and the joint can be damaged (*chronic arthritis*).

Heart disease can develop with irregular heart rhythm (*carditis*).

The central nervous system can be affected as well. Meningitis can develop with symptoms of fever, vomiting, lethargy, and stiff neck (see *neck pain, stiff neck*).

Palsy of the facial nerve (*Bell's palsy*) is common. If the child has Bell's palsy, the corner of the mouth drops, and he or she is unable to close the eye on the affected side. If your child has these symptoms, see the doctor as soon as possible, or go to the emergency room. An eye doctor is often involved with the child's care, because the eye that does not close can get very dry, and eye damage can be the consequence.

Diagnosis of Lyme disease is made by history of the tick bite if it is known, the specific rash if it is present, the clinical picture, and laboratory tests. However, the laboratory tests by themselves do not make the diagnosis. Early diagnosis is important to start the treatment early.

Treatment: Remove the tick completely with a tweezer as soon as possible.

Antibiotics

Prevention: Always have your child wear a long sleeve shirt and long pants, closed shoes, and a hat when going to the woods.

Learning disorders or learning disabilities

Learning disorder means that the child has difficulty learning. It can affect one or more subjects.

Learning disorders can make it difficult for the child to learn reading, writing, or math.

Dyslexia is a learning disorder in reading.

Children with learning disorders have difficulty understanding how letters can represent sounds and how they become words.

They also have problem understanding what they read, and it is difficult for them to recall it.

They also have trouble with spelling.

The writing is slow and difficult and hard to read. They might also have problem with drawing and cutting with scissors.

In math, they have a problem understanding how the numbers work and how to calculate. This is called *dyscalculia.*

They might have problems with nonverbal communication, like interpreting facial expression.

Motor coordination can be problematic as well.

Some children struggle in school before the diagnosis of learning disorder is made, and that can affect their self-esteem and motivation. They can be frustrated and act out.

Early intervention is most important.

These children need evaluation, and that includes hearing and vision tests.

Treatment:

- Tutoring.
- Classroom accommodation.
- Individualized education program.
- If the child has problem with motor skills, occupational therapy (OT) and/or physical therapy (PT) can help.
- Children who also have attention deficit hyperactivity disorder (ADHD) often need medication.

If your child struggle in school and has more difficulty with reading, writing, or math than other children of the same age, see the doctor.

The parents, the doctor, other health professionals, and the school work together to do the testing and find the best treatment for the child.

Lice (pediculosis)

Head lice is the most common type of lice. It is a small parasite that sometimes can be seen by the naked eye. Head lice is the most common cause of head itching. It is contagious and can cause school outbreaks. Head lice spreads from person to person by close contact (from hair to hair), but brushes and combs can also transmit the lice. Intense head itching raises the suspicion that the child has lice. Nits (tiny whitish bulbs) can be seen on the hair shafts. The nits are strongly attached to the hair shaft, so it is not easy to remove them. The presence of nits confirms that the child has head lice. Dandruff is the shedding of small pieces of dead skin from the scalp. Dandruff can look similar to nits, but it easily comes off from the hair.

Medicated shampoos and lotions help to eliminate head lice. You can get some of these medications over the counter like Nix shampoo, but some are prescriptions like Ovide shampoo. The nits need to be removed in order to get rid of the head lice. A special fine-tooth comb is used. The combs and brushes of the child who had head lice should be sterilized. Clothing has to be washed. After treatment, the hair needs to be checked regularly for several days to be sure that there is no recurrence. All household members and other close contacts should be checked and treated if nits or lice are found. Do not use regular shampoo or conditioner before using lice medicine, and do not wash the hair again for two days after the lice medicine is removed.

The best treatment is prevention. Teach your child not to share brushes and combs.

There are two other types of lice—*body lice and crab lice (pubic lice)*.

In case of body lice, the nits stick to the clothes. Body lice can cause a serious disease, typhus (see typhus).

Pubic lice are attached to pubic hair. It spreads through sexual contact.

Good hygiene can prevent both body and pubic lice.

Menstrual period (menstrual cycle), menstrual problems

The normal menstrual cycle occurs every twenty-one to forty-five days. It lasts less than seven days and not more than three to six pads are used per day.

Keep a menstrual calendar that shows the date of the last period and the length of the cycle.

Menstrual periods can be irregular in the first year. But if the irregularity continues, tell to the doctor.

If there is a delay of a period, see the doctor.

Avoid the use of tampons to prevent a serious disease called *toxic shock syndrome.* The cause is toxins produced by germs, namely, *Staphylococcus* or group A *Streptococcus.* Symptoms are high fever, headache, vomiting or diarrhea, rash, low blood pressure, muscle pain, and seizure. Toxic shock syndrome can affect multiple organs. Treatment includes antibiotics, fluids, and medications for low blood pressure. Surgery may be necessary (removal of infected tissue).

Severe cramps or dysmenorrhea

Important questions:

- How severe is the pain?
- Is there any fever or vaginal discharge?
- Is there a family history of severe menstrual pain?

Treatment is usually ibuprofen.

If the pain is severe or accompanied by other symptoms as well, your daughter needs to see the doctor.

The lack of menstrual periods or amenorrhea. If there is no sign of sexual development and the adolescent girl never had a period by sixteen years of age, she has so-called primary amenorrhea. In this case, there is a suspicion of a genetic problem called Turner's syndrome. Genetic testing is needed to make the diagnosis.

In so-called secondary amenorrhea, after having regular periods, there is an absence of menstruation, at least three cycles.

There can be many causes of secondary amenorrhea, like extremely vigorous exercise, extreme dieting, thyroid problem, pregnancy, etc. Laboratory tests are needed, including a pregnancy test to find the cause. In any case, the doctor needs to be seen.

If there are fewer than eight cycles a year, the condition is called *oligomenorrhea.*

Heavy menstrual bleeding or menorrhagia. There are different causes of abnormal flow.

One cause is that the egg is not released during the cycle like it is supposed to be. Family history is important. A bleeding disorder can be another cause. Laboratory tests are needed to make the diagnosis.

The doctor needs to be seen.

Uterine bleeding at irregular intervals or metrorrhagia. The bleeding occurs in between regular menstrual periods.

See the doctor to look for the cause.

Usually a gynecologist is involved in the management of these disorders.

Methemoglobulinemia.

Methemoglobinemia is a condition when methemoglobin is elevated in the blood. Normally, hemoglobin in the red blood cells carries oxygen to the organs of the body. In case of methemoglobinemia, the hemoglobin changes, becomes dysfunctional, and cannot carry oxygen. Some substances can cause methemoglobinemia, like nitrates, benzocaine, and aniline.

Symptoms depend on the amount of methemoglobin, because the more methemoglobin is in the blood, the less amount of oxygen is available for the body.

The baby looks blue, and in severe cases, trouble breathing and loss of consciousness can develop. If your baby looks blue, call 911.

Treatment is methylene blue injected into the vein.

Prevention is important. Carrots and well water can contain nitrates. Do not prepare your own carrots. Buy the jar instead. Do not give well water to your baby. Do not use benzocaine for numbing your baby's gum if teething or hurt if he is younger than two years old. If your child is older and you use benzocaine, be sure he does not swallow it. Prevent aniline poisoning. Aniline is present in dyes, varnishes, herbicides, etc.

Mononucleosis (mono)

Mononucleosis is a viral illness, caused by the Epstein-Barr virus (EB virus).

The incubation period is thirty to fifty days. It is moderately contagious.

The symptoms are fever for several days, sore throat, often tonsillitis, and enlarged lymph nodes on the neck. The spleen and liver can also be enlarged, and the child is tired all the time. Rash can develop, but mostly after the child took amoxicillin for the sore throat. A child also can have mononucleosis and strep throat at the same time. The doctor needs to see the sick child.

The diagnosis is made by blood tests. Monospot is a screening test. A blood count is done that includes the so-called blood smear. This test can support the diagnosis. EB virus antibodies can be detected in the blood, and that confirms the diagnosis.

The disease can last for weeks. Hepatitis can develop.

Treatment: There is no specific treatment for mononucleosis. Give ibuprofen to treat the fever. Do not use Tylenol, because that can affect the liver.

It is important not to play contact sports for three to four weeks and until the spleen is not enlarged anymore to prevent spleen rupture. Regular follow-up with the doctor is necessary.

Mosquito-transmitted diseases

These are malaria, dengue fever, chikungunya, West Nile virus, Zika virus. People traveling to areas where these diseases are common are at risk of infection.

Malaria. Malaria is a very serious disease caused by a protozoa (plasmodium), a microscopic-size parasite.

The incubation period is seven to thirty days.

There are four types of plasmodiums that can cause the disease.

It is common in India and parts of Africa.

Symptoms are recurrent high fever, chills, anemia, and enlarged spleen and liver. The central nervous system, lung, and kidneys can also be involved.

Diagnosis is made by blood test, looking for the parasites.

Patients have relapses after recovering from the first attack.

Medications are available for treatment. They are also used for prevention, like mefloquine. If your child travels to areas where malaria is common, medication needs to be taken, so talk to the doctor. The first dose is usually started two weeks before departure, and the last dose is taken four weeks after return.

A malaria vaccine was developed recently (RTS,S).

Dengue fever. It is caused by a virus.

It is present in different parts of the world, but the closest locations to the USA are the Caribbean, Central America, and South America. Few cases occur in the USA.

Symptoms are fever, headache, muscle and joint pain, and rash. If the disease is severe, it can cause respiratory distress, severe bleeding, and organ damage.

The diagnosis is made by a blood test.

After a previous dengue infection, there is a higher risk of having a severe disease from the dengue virus.

No specific treatment is available.

Prevention: a vaccine is available to prevent dengue fever, called Dengvaxia. This shot is recommended for children aged nine to sixteen if they have evidence of a previous dengue infection and live in an area where dengue fever is common (epidemic).

A previous dengue infection should be confirmed by lab tests before the shot is given, otherwise the child can get a severe form of the disease if he gets the dengue virus after getting the shot.

Chikungunya disease. It is caused by a virus. It is present in different parts of the world, but the closest locations to the USA are the Caribbean and South America. Few cases occur in the USA.

Symptoms are fever, muscle ache, joint swelling, headache, and rash. Joint pain can continue even after the disease is over.

The diagnosis is made by a blood test.

No specific treatment is available.

Zika virus infection. Zika virus gained publicity in recent years.

It is present in South America, Central America, and the Caribbean. A few cases occurred in Florida.

Many people infected with Zika virus have no symptoms at all or only mild symptoms.

Symptoms are fever, rash, joint pain, pink eye (conjunctivitis), muscle pain, headache.

The disease is very dangerous for pregnant women because it may harm the fetus. Newborns may have severe deformities, very small head and brain (microcephaly), that cause mental deficiencies (see large, small, misshapen head).

The diagnosis is made by blood or urine test.

No specific treatment is available.

Pregnant women should not travel to places where Zika virus is common.

West Nile virus disease. It is caused by a virus.

It is present in different parts of the world, including the Southern United States.

Symptoms are fever, muscle pain (myalgia), headache, weakness, often abdominal pain, vomiting, and diarrhea. Neurologic problems like inflammation of the brain (encephalitis) or infection of the membrane around the brain (aseptic meningitis) are the most serious manifestations of the disease. In that case, lethargy, headache, vomiting, stiff neck, muscle weakness, sometimes seizures are the symptoms.

The diagnosis is made by blood test.

No specific treatment is available.

Japanese encephalitis and yellow fever. These are also caused by viruses transmitted by mosquitoes. These diseases are mostly present in certain parts of Asia and Africa. Preventive shots are available. Travelers who visit those countries where the diseases occur are required to get the shots.

Prevention is important in all of the diseases caused by mosquitoes. Avoid being outside from dusk to dawn, when most of the bites happen.

Keep your skin covered with protective clothing (long-sleeve shirt, pan, long socks, and a hat).

Use mosquito repellents. Repellents with DEET are the most effective.

Read and follow all directions and precautions on the product label.

The repellent should be applied only by an adult. Keep it out of reach of children.

Do not use a sunscreen and bug spray combination because sunscreens need to be reapplied regularly.

In infested areas, nets impregnated with insecticide can be used. Sleep under the net.

Do not leave outside hoses dripping because mosquitoes like wet, damp places.

Motion sickness

Motion sickness develops when the child goes on any kind of transportation or rides at an amusement park.

He feels uneasy, gets dizzy, and may vomit.

Here are some advices to avoid motion sickness:

- Have your child look straight ahead in the car, and keep his head still, resting against the back of the seat.
- Avoid making sharp turns with the car or boat.
- Prefer forward-facing seat on trains and midship cabins on ships.
- Sit in the front of the airplane before the wings.

If your child has significant motion sickness, talk to the doctor since medications are available.

Muscle pain

Muscle pain can be caused by injury, inflammation, and overuse of the muscle.

The pain can be local and generalized. It can be regular pain or cramps.

Children can have *growing pain*. It affects both legs and can be experienced at night. If the pain is recurrent, see the doctor. However, if the pain is consistent, getting worse, affects the joints, or only one leg is involved, the child needs to see the doctor soon.

Cramps often develop after the child plays sports, and it is most commonly from muscle strain.

Gentle massage can help.

Dehydration and low blood calcium level also can cause muscle cramps.

If the child has frequent or consistent muscle cramps, see the doctor.

Treatment is called RICE: rest, ice, compression, elevation.

Rest is needed to provide healing time after the injury. If there is no improvement after one or two days, visit the doctor. If the pain is strong or if any deformity is present, go to the emergency room. If the foot, ankle, or legs are very swollen, painful, and the child cannot put weight on that leg, do not wait. Go to the emergency room. If the child cannot walk, have him or her use crutches.

Ice should be used intermittently, not longer than twenty minutes at a time. Be sure to wrap the ice in a towel or cloth so it does not touch the skin directly.

Compression: An elastic bandage can be used. Be sure that it is not too tight so the skin color does not change.

Elevation of the extremity is helpful in decreasing swelling.

If the pain is significant, Tylenol or ibuprofen can be given.

Inflammation of the muscle (myositis) can occur with viral infections.

Influenza virus often causes body ache, when most of the muscles hurt.

If the muscle gets hit very hard, the contusion can cause bleeding inside the muscle. The accumulated blood becomes hard from calcification (*myositis ossificans*). If this hard area is large, it can cause functional problems. Usually orthopedic consultation is necessary.

Bleeding disorders like hemophilia can cause bleeding to the muscle even after small trauma. (See bleeding disorders.)

Muscle strain

Muscle strain is an injury to a muscle or a tendon (pulled muscle). Tendons connect muscles to bones.

Muscle strain is often caused by a sports injury.

Symptoms are pain, tenderness, bruising, muscle spasms, and limited motion.

Treatment is RICE: rest, ice, compression, elevation, like in the case of muscle pain.

No sports.

Use the ice for fifteen to twenty minutes every two to three hours. Do not put it directly to the skin.

For compression, use an elastic bandage. Be sure it is not too tight.

For elevation, you can use pillows.

Tylenol or ibuprofen can help the pain.

The use of crutches may be necessary.

If the symptoms do not improve in a couple of days, they are severe or getting worse, see the doctor. If your child has numbness or tingling, go to the emergency room.

In case of a severe muscle strain, usually an orthopedic specialist participates in the child's care.

Maybe a brace or splint is needed to immobilize the area.

In case of a torn tendon or torn muscle, surgery can be necessary.

Be sure that your child does not go back to sports too soon.

Prevention is stretching and strengthening exercises before sports.

Muscle weakness

Different diseases and disorders can cause muscle weakness. They can affect the brain, spine, nerves, and muscles.

Decreased muscle tone (hypotonia). The resistance to stretch the muscle is low. It occurs with muscle atrophy and dystrophy. It can be congenital or develop later. It can be discovered after birth, during infancy, or childhood.

The baby can be floppy, not performing age-appropriate motor functions, like holding his or her head, rolling over, sitting up, and walking. Children can have a problem scribbling, drawing, and using scissors.

But also it can be a regression of the motor functions, like in case of *Duchenne muscular dystrophy.* Respiratory and heart problems are also frequent in that disease.

Myasthenia gravis. The characteristic feature of this rare muscle disease is unusual fatigability of the muscles. The child is okay after waking up, but the muscles are getting weaker and weaker with daily activities.

Treatment is available (anticholinesterase drugs).

There are also the so-called *myotonic muscle diseases,* where after a muscle contraction, the relaxation is delayed.

Poliomyelitis (Polio). Poliomyelitis is an infectious disease caused by a virus. It is transmitted from person to person, and mainly affects children younger than five.

Symptoms are fever, fatigue, headache, vomiting, stiff neck, muscle weakness. But paralysis and trouble breathing and swallowing are the most severe symptoms.

No specific treatment is available.

Prevention: Vaccination is the best way to prevent polio. The immunization schedule includes the polio vaccine (IPV).

Thanks to vaccinations, polio has been eradicated in most countries, including the USA.

Acute flaccid myelitis (AFM). This is a serious but rare disease of the spinal cord.

The condition mainly affects young children. Usually the child has a mild respiratory illness (viral infection) before the symptoms develop.

The cause of acute flaccid myelitis is unknown.

It is a sudden weakness of the limbs. Reflexes get weak as well. The child also can have problems moving his face, swallowing, and breathing. The diagnosis is made by the clinical picture. MRI is also helpful.

Spinal tap and examination of the cerebrospinal fluid helps to rule out other causes.

Urgent medical care is necessary. Go to the emergency room, or call 911.

No specific treatment is available, but intravenous (into the vein) immunoglobulin (IVIG) has been used. Early physical and occupational therapy is important.

Guillain-Barré syndrome. Guillain-Barré syndrome is a rare disorder.

The first symptoms are usually weakness and tingling in both legs. Then it spreads to the upper body and can lead to paralysis.

Urgent medical care is necessary. Go to the emergency room.

No specific treatment is available.

Suddenly developing muscle weakness is always an emergency. Go to the emergency room or call 911.

A neurologist participates in the child's care.

Treatment is symptomatic.

Neck pain, stiff neck

Neck pain can be caused by different conditions.

Many diseases, bacterial or viral, can cause enlarged, painful, tender lymph nodes in the neck. Pain and swelling in front of the ears are characteristic of mumps (see infectious diseases of childhood).

The neck can be painful and stiff from trauma. If significant neck injury is suspected, do not move the child, keep him or her on the floor, hold the head still, and call 911.

Slight trauma of the neck muscle (sternocleidomastoid) or muscle strain of the same muscle can cause pain and stiff neck. The head leans to one side and cannot be straightened out because of the pain. The condition is called *torticollis*. In children, it is usually caused by sleeping in the wrong position or by a sudden movement in the wrong way. Treatment is rest and pain medicine like ibuprofen or Tylenol if needed. It usually resolves after three to four days. But if the torticollis is secondary to neck injury, x-ray of the neck is often necessary. Torticollis sometimes also can be noted after birth. Then usually a small lump can be felt on the neck muscle. The treatment of torticollis after birth is physiotherapy.

If the child has a stiff neck, fever, headache, vomiting, and lethargy, infection of the membranes around the brain (*meningitis*) or another problem in the central nervous system is suspected (see vomiting). In case of meningitis, the neck cannot be moved up and down. If the child has torticollis, only the side movements are restricted secondary to the pain.

Stiff neck should always be considered as a severe symptom.

If the child has neck pain or stiffness of the neck, medical care is necessary. However, if meningitis is suspected, go to the emergency room right away, or call 911.

Nose bleeding

Nosebleeds are frequent during childhood.

Nose picking, scratching, injury, and strong nose blowing are the most common causes.

Children sometimes push a foreign body into their nostril, and that can cause nosebleeds as well.

Nose blowing usually causes nosebleeds when the child has a cold (upper respiratory infection).

Scratching is often caused by itching secondary to allergies.

Important questions:

- When was the nosebleed?
- How strong was the bleeding?
- How long did it last?
- How was it stopped?
- Is this the first time the child had a nosebleed? If not, how often did it happen?
- Does the child pick his or her nose?
- Does the child put things in his or her nose?
- Did the child have a cold?
- Does he or she have allergies?
- Does he or she get bruises easily?
- Is there anybody in the family who has a bleeding problem?

When you want to stop the nosebleed, apply pressure from the side of the nose all the way to the bone for at least five minutes. When the bleeding stops, release the pressure gradually. If the bleeding recurs regularly, put saline nose drops and/or Vaseline into the nostrils to decrease dryness there, because that also can lead to bleeding. Do not lay the child down because he or she can swallow the blood. Vomiting up the swallowed blood is not uncommon.

If the child has nosebleeds that are hard to control and gets bruises easily, a bleeding disorder should be suspected. If the nosebleed was hard to stop or it is frequently recurring, medical attention is needed. Severe unstoppable nosebleed is an emergency. Go to the emergency room, or call 911.

In case of severe and frequently recurring nosebleeds, often a consultation with an ear, nose, and throat (ENT) specialist is arranged. If pressure has not stopped the bleeding, packing of the nose with gauze can be necessary. If the bleeding frequently recurs, the child may need cauterization. A chemical, silver nitrate, is used to burn the blood vessel that caused the bleeding. Sometimes electrocautery is used.

To prevent recurring nosebleeds, petroleum jelly is applied inside the nose.

Frequent nosebleeds can cause anemia. A simple laboratory test, blood count (CBC), can detect it.

Obesity

Many times when a child is significantly overweight, parents think that it is caused by an illness. But that is rarely the case. Decreased function of the thyroid gland (hypothyroidism) can cause it, as well as a few rare diseases. However, most of the time, it is caused by overeating and inactivity. The weight depends on the calorie intake and the calorie burning. It is important to have a good balance between the calories taken in as food and the calories burned by activities.

Obesity means that the child's Body Mass Index (BMI) is over 30 (overweight is over 25) on the growth chart. The doctor checks the child's BMI.

Children, like adults, often prefer foods that are high in calories, such as pizza, pasta, tortilla, fried foods, sweets, and junk food. They also like to drink sodas and other sweet drinks high in calories. Lately, children spend more time in front of the TV and playing video games than ever. It is not rare that they spend three to four hours a day or even more with these activities. No wonder so many children are overweight.

Obesity can lead to health problems, like diabetes, high blood pressure, high cholesterol, fatty liver, and breathing problems from sleep apnea. If a child has sleep apnea, then he or she stops breathing for a few seconds when sleeping, several times a night. That can lead to heart problems as well (cor pulmonale).

High cholesterol and high blood pressure can also cause heart problems.

The body contains fat (lipids) in the form of *triglycerides* and *cholesterol.*

In obese children, the triglycerides and cholesterol need to be checked. The name of the blood test is lipid profile, and the child needs to fast before the test. When checking the cholesterol, the test shows the total cholesterol, the "good" cholesterol or high-density lipoprotein (HDL cholesterol), and the "bad" cholesterol or low density lipoprotein (LDL cholesterol). High LDL cholesterol level increases the risk of heart problems (coronary artery disease).

High triglyceride and cholesterol level can be inherited, so let the doctor know about your family history. It is important to know if any family member has had a problem with high cholesterol or triglycerides. But an unhealthy diet containing much fat and carbohydrates also can cause high levels.

Foods containing high cholesterol are red meat, eggs, cheese, and coconut and palm oil.

Foods containing high carbohydrates are sugar, pasta, pizza, tortilla, bread, and potato.

If the lipid profile test shows high total cholesterol, low HDL cholesterol, and high LDL cholesterol, that means that the child has predisposition for early heart disease from hardening of the blood vessels.

The treatment is a diet rich in vegetables, fruits, fibers, fish, and chicken but containing less red meat, eggs, and cheese. Eating salmon can increase the "good" cholesterol (HDL cholesterol).

If the diet does not solve the problem, and the numbers are high, medications can be used. Often a cardiologist is consulted. In case of extreme obesity, the so-called bariatric surgery can be necessary to help the child lose weight.

Obesity also contributes to the development of orthopedic problems, such as the hip problem called slipped capital femoral epiphysis—when the head of the thigh bone (femur) is displaced. Obesity also predisposes to the development of bow legs and flat feet (see flatfoot and other orthopedic problems).

Obesity can cause low self-esteem, social isolation, and depression.

Obesity often starts early on. An obese toddler will probably be an obese adult.

Therefore, it is important not to feed a baby right away when he or she starts to cry, if the last feeding was only a short while ago. Do not let the baby have the bottle all the time. Food is not supposed to be a pacifier. Also, children should not be pushed to finish all the food that is in front of them. Do not let your child eat all the time. Some children like to snack all day long. Have regular family meals.

Teach your child to eat a well-balanced diet, including all the vegetables and fruits.

Teach your child not to eat all the candies and ice cream he or she has at once, not even on Halloween, but save them for another day.

Limit the time your child spends in front of the TV or playing video games. Instead, encourage physical activities and sports. If a child is overweight, these measures are even more important. If your child is overweight, you also need to limit portions of foods that are high in calories, including bread. You want to substitute them with vegetables and fruits so your child will not be hungry. The intake of junk food needs to be limited. Also limit the amount of sweet drinks, including sodas. Even fruit juice should not be more than four to eight ounces a day. Your child can still eat all kinds of foods, but less from those containing high calories.

If you go to the doctor because your child is overweight, take a diary with you, showing what he or she was eating during the past two to four weeks, and include the amounts.

Pets can transmit diseases to children

Cat scratch disease. This can develop if the child gets a cat scratch or bite. Symptoms are fever, malaise, headache, and enlarged lymph nodes (see cat scratch disease).

Leptospirosis. Leptospirosis is a bacterial disease. Leptospira is an organism that is excreted in animal urine, including dogs.

Children can get it through contaminated soil or water. Incubation period is five to fourteen days.

Symptoms are fever, headache, muscle ache, vomiting, and pink eye. Severe disease such as meningitis can develop as well (see vomiting).

Diagnosis is made from blood samples.

Treatment is antibiotic therapy.

Lymphocytic choriomeningitis. Lymphocytic choriomeningitis is a viral disease. It can be transmitted to a child by a pet hamster.

The child can have the symptoms of meningitis, like fever, vomiting, lethargy (see vomiting), or other neurologic signs and symptoms.

There is no specific therapy.

Pasteurella infections. Pasteurella is a bacterial infection. The germ lives in the saliva of dogs and cats.

The incubation period is less than twenty-four hours.

Skin infection, cellulitis (see skin infections), is frequent at the site of the bite, scratch, or licking of a dog or cat, causing redness, swelling, and tenderness in the area. Local lymph nodes can get infected and enlarged. Skin abscess, infection of the joint (septic arthritis), or a bone (osteomyelitis) can develop. Less frequently, other organs, the brain, lung, and heart can be affected, so meningitis, pneumonia, and endocarditis can develop.

Treatment is antibiotics.

Salmonella infections. This can be caused by chickens, ducks, reptiles, and turtles (see diarrhea).

Psittacosis. Psittacosis is a bacterial infection spread by birds such as parrots.

Incubation period is five to fifteen days.

Symptoms are fever, cough, muscle pain, and malaise. The most common disease caused by psittacosis is pneumonia.

Treatment is antibiotic therapy.

Rabies. (See bites.)

Worms

Ascariasis. Ascaris lumbricoides is a roundworm.

Children can get it by ingesting eggs from contaminated soil. The eggs get to the soil from human and animal waste.

Symptoms are abdominal discomfort, nausea, malnutrition. But symptoms of pneumonia or even bowel obstruction can develop as well.

Hookworm—cutaneous larva migrans. The larvae of cat and dog hookworms cause a very itchy reddish bump on the skin and migrate through the skin. Rarely it can penetrate deeper tissues. Children can get it if they are in contact with soil contaminated with dog or cat feces (walking barefoot). The disease is usually self-limited after weeks or months. Antiparasitic drugs like Albendazole can help.

Tapeworm and trichinellosis. Children get infected if they eat incompletely cooked meat.

Both diseases can cause nausea, diarrhea, and stomachache. But they also can cause severe diseases when the larvae get to the bloodstream and reach different organs.

The severe form of tapeworm is called *cysticercosis* and that affects the nervous system. It can cause seizures and hydrocephalus (see head: large, small, misshapen).

Trichinellosis can cause heart disease (myocarditis), pneumonia, and neurologic problems.

Both diseases are treated with different kinds of medications.

Toxocariasis. Toxocara or roundworms are parasitic diseases (a parasite is an organism that lives in a host and gets food from the host).

These roundworms come from dogs or, less commonly, from cats. Puppies are often infected.

Infected dogs and cats shed Toxocara eggs in their feces to the soil. These eggs can survive for months or years. Humans and animals can get infected by accidentally ingesting the eggs. When in the body, the eggs hatch, and the larvae can travel in the bloodstream to different organs like the liver, heart, lungs, brain, muscles, or eyes. This condition is called visceral toxocariasis or visceral larva migrans. The symptoms depend on the affected organs. The child can have pneumonia or an enlarged liver, since the Toxocara can damage those organs. However, most infected people have no symptoms.

Children with worms can be asymptomatic or have a mild or severe disease.

The diagnosis is made from stool samples.

Treatment is anthelmintic (antiparasitic) drugs like albendazole or mebendazole.

Prevention is very important.

Have the veterinarian treat your dogs and cats regularly for worms.

Clean your pet's living area daily.

Do not allow children to play in soiled areas.

Be sure that your child's hands are thoroughly cleaned with warm water and soap after playing with your pet. He or she needs to learn early on that handwashing is absolutely necessary before touching any food.

Teach your child not to eat any dirt or soil, because it is dangerous.

Toxoplasmosis. The newborn can get infected from the mother if she was exposed to infected cat feces.

Therefore, pregnant women should not change cat litter (see agents that can harm the fetus).

Prevention:

- Keep your pet's vaccinations up to date.
- Have regular checkups with the veterinarian.
- Have your pet only eat and drink from his dish.
- Clean cat litter boxes daily, but pregnant women should not touch it.

Pinworms

The most common intestinal parasites in the US are pinworms. Pinworms are small, white, threadlike worms.

Parents often get frightened when they see pinworms, often moving in the baby's or child's stool.

Some parents take their child to the emergency room when they find pinworms. This is unnecessary since pinworms are not dangerous. But they cause itching of the rectum at night, disturbing the sleep.

In girls, pinworms can cause itching at the genital area and vaginal discharge.

Pinworms can be passed from child to child if they share contaminated objects.

The best diagnostic test is to look at the stools and actually see the pinworms.

If no pinworm is seen but there is a strong suspicion that the child has pinworms because of rectal or vaginal itching, the diagnosis can be made by a laboratory test. The most efficient test is to place a piece of scotch tape to the rectal area. The tape will be checked in the lab for eggs.

The best prevention is good handwashing.

Keep the child in long pajamas, not too loose, to make it harder for him to scratch the rectum at night, when female worms come out and lay eggs at the rectum, causing the itching. Be sure to cut the fingernails short to prevent reinfection. Namely, when the child scratches the rectum, eggs get under the fingernails, and when he or she puts the hand in the mouth, reinfection occurs.

Treatment: Contaminated objects should be sterilized by hot water, and the bedding should be washed. The doctor can give your child medication, like mebendazole or albendazole. Usually a second dose is given, and the whole family is treated at the same time to eradicate the infection.

Poisoning

The best treatment is prevention. Make your house poison-proof. Check the areas where poisonous substances are kept.

Keep all medications and chemicals locked all the time. Some parents put these substances on the top shelf so their child cannot reach them. But that is still not safe.

One day the child will discover that he or she can take a chair there, stand on it, and reach the top shelf. Be sure that if you take out something poisonous, you put it back in the safe place.

Always read the labels, and learn if any substance in your home is poisonous.

Have the Poison Control Center's telephone number readily available (1-800-222-1222).

The most common hazardous products are medications, including aspirin, alcohol, methyl alcohol, antifreeze, cleaning and polishing agents (furniture polish), pesticides, fertilizers, insecticides, hydrocarbons, petrolatum distillates (Kerosene) paint thinner, charcoal starter, turpentine, acids, lyes like ammonia, carbon monoxide from cars, and fuels kept at home or in the garage.

Parents often have suspicions when their child ingested something poisonous.

Important questions:

- Why do you think your child ingested a poisonous substance?
- Did you find a bottle with medication or chemical close to your child?
- Was the bottle open?
- Was anything missing from the bottle? If it was medicine, how many tablets were in the bottle, and how many left? If it was a chemical, did you see it on the clothing of your child? Did you smell any odor on the clothes or in your child's breath?
- Was your child gagging, coughing, choking, or drooling? Has he or she had any problem swallowing?

- Did you see any sore on the skin or in the mouth?

The symptoms can be general, occurring with many illnesses, or specific to a certain poison.

Some common poisonings

Poisoning from medications. Among the medications, acetaminophen (Tylenol) often causes poisoning because it is one of the most often used medicines. Until the recent past, Tylenol drops were often used. These drops were much more concentrated than the liquid form. Therefore, when the same amount of medicine was given from the drops accidentally, as it would be the liquid, sometimes poisoning occurred. One teaspoonful or 5 milliliters of Tylenol liquid and 0.8 milliliter of Tylenol drops equally contained one hundred milligrams of Tylenol.

That is the reason why the drops are not available in pharmacies anymore.

Large amounts of Tylenol ingestion (acute poisoning) can cause liver damage. In the emergency room, the blood level of acetaminophen is taken. Four hours after the ingestion occurred, it is best to check the blood level. That will show how much medicine was taken and therefore how dangerous the poisoning is and how it should be treated.

But even if the regular dose of Tylenol is given for a long time (chronic poisoning), liver damage can develop.

Another frequently used fever reducer and painkiller is Ibuprofen (Motrin, Advil, etc.) It can cause kidney damage if a large dose is taken or if it is used for a long time.

Antihistamines (Benadryl, Claritin, Zyrtec, Allegra, etc.) and atropine poisoning cause similar symptoms. These symptoms are dry mouth, flushed skin, dilated pupils, blurred vision, and fast heartbeats.

Aspirin poisoning (salicylate poisoning)
Symptoms: fever, fast heartbeats and breathing, sweating, vomiting, diarrhea, dehydration, convulsions, and coma can occur. There is low blood sugar in younger children (see sweating, hunger, trembling).

If there is a suspicion of salicylate poisoning, go to the emergency room or call 911.

Barbiturates. These cause drowsiness, a problem with thinking, and the fall of blood pressure.

Opiates. (Morphine, heroin, meperidine, methadone, fentanyl, hydrocodone, codeine, and many other strong painkillers.)
Symptoms are slow breathing, very small so-called pinpoint pupils, and the fall of blood pressure. These drugs are not recommended for children, only under very special circumstances. Be sure your child cannot get ahold of this kind of medicine because any of these medications can cause a life-threatening condition and death if a large amount of medicine is taken. Fentanyl is particularly dangerous because it is very potent. Treatment is Naloxone.

Clonidine. Clonidine poisoning symptoms are similar to those seen in opioid poisoning.

Tricyclic antidepressant poisoning (imipramine, amitriptyline, desipramine, nortriptyline)
Symptoms are lethargy, fast heartbeats, flushed dry skin, low blood pressure, and the pupils are wider than usual. These drugs can affect the heart muscles and the nervous system, and they can cause seizures and coma.

Birth control pills. These can cause vomiting, but vaginal bleeding can occur too.

Vitamin overdose (hypervitaminosis). If a child gets more vitamin A or D than the recommended dose, that also can be harmful.
Excessive dose of vitamin A (acute hypervitaminosis A) can cause symptoms like vomiting, drowsiness, double vision. These are signs of increased pressure inside the head (increased intracranial pressure). This condition is called *pseudotumor cerebri*. In babies, the soft spot is bulging.

If a higher dose is given for a longer time (chronic hypervitaminosis A), loss of appetite, lack of weight gain, irritability, itching, tenderness, and swelling of the bones can be the consequence.

Ingestion of *excessive dose of vitamin D* (hypervitaminosis D) can cause symptoms of lack of appetite, irritability, decreased muscle tone, and constipation. Thirst and large amounts of daily urine with kidney damage can also be seen.

Excessive iron intake can cause bloody vomiting and diarrhea. Shock can develop as well. (See change in consciousness, fast breathing, cold sweat, shock.)

If your child has any of these symptoms, see the doctor. But with severe symptoms, go to the emergency room, or call 911.

Diazepam (Valium) poisoning
Symptoms: drowsiness, confusion, slurred speech, incoordination, but severe poisoning can cause coma or stop breathing.

If overdose is suspected, go to the emergency room, or call 911.

Poisoning from chemicals

All of these substances can cause life-threatening conditions.

Acids. Acid can be found in certain fertilizers, pool chemicals, and toilet cleaners.

It causes burning on contact.

Symptoms after a child swallowed acid: drooling and burning sensation inside the mouth and esophagus. Other symptoms are severe abdominal pain, problem speaking, and difficulty breathing. Coughing, chest pain, and bloody vomiting are also in the picture. Shock can develop as well.

Treatment: Do not make the child vomit. Call 911.

Alkali. Many household products contain alkali, like drain cleaner and laundry bleaches.

Symptoms are drooling, burning sensation in the mouth, vomiting, often bloody, and problems swallowing (dysphagia). Other symptoms are coughing, fast and heavy breathing, chest and stomach pain, and problem speaking.

Alkali poisoning can cause narrowing of the esophagus and perforation.

Treatment: Do not make the child vomit. Call 911.

Acids and lyes can cause narrowing of the esophagus, constriction, or even stricture.

Alcohol (ethanol). All the alcohols can be toxic. Metanol, ethylene glycol (see below), and isopropyl alcohol are very dangerous. Ethanol, regularly called alcohol, is the only type of alcohol people can drink, but even that can cause poisoning.

Symptoms are blurred vision, unsteady gait, slurred speech. Drinking alcohol before driving is particularly dangerous.

If the mother is a chronic alcohol user, the baby can be born with fetal alcohol syndrome (see alcohol, drug use disorder, and tobacco use of the mother).

Methanol. Products that contain methanol are home-distilled spirits, windshield washer fluid, household solvents, cooking fuels, printing ink, and perfumes.

Methanol is very toxic to children, even in very small amounts.

Symptoms are headache, nausea, vomiting, abdominal pain, clumsiness, blurry vision, and blindness. But methanol also can cause heart, lung, and kidney problems. Seizures and coma can develop as well.

Treatment is fomepizole.

Arsenic. Symptoms are metallic taste, hoarseness, difficulty swallowing, and dehydration. Chronic poisoning can cause weight loss, vomiting, bloody diarrhea, and kidney damage.

Carbon monoxide. Carbon monoxide is a colorless, odorless, gas produced by burning gasoline, woods, coal, etc. in an enclosed space. If a child inhales carbon monoxide, that creates a dangerous, life-threatening situation.

Symptoms are headache, weakness, dizziness, confusion, vomiting, blurred vision, problem breathing, loss of consciousness.

If there is a suspicion of carbon monoxide poisoning, take the child into fresh air, and call 911.

Naturally fix the problem that caused the poisoning in the first place.

Prevention:

- Appropriate use of appliances
- Proper ventilation
- Carbon monoxide detector

Ethylene glycol. Ethylene glycol is an odorless, sweet substance found in antifreeze products.

It is very dangerous and life-threatening for children.

Symptoms are drowsiness, stumbling around like a drunk, slurred speech, lethargy, and seizures. Fast breathing, bluish discoloration of the lips, face, fingernails, heart failure, shock, and coma develop. Acute renal failure can develop as well.

If ethylene glycol poisoning is suspected, call 911.

Lead poisoning. The main source of lead exposure is paint containing lead and dust that contains lead.

Acute lead poisoning

Symptoms: persistent vomiting, weakness, irritability, ataxia (see jerking and strange movements), and altered consciousness. Lead poisoning can lead to seizures and coma.

Chronic lead poisoning causes developmental delay and regression and intellectual disability. It also can cause personality change, abdominal pain, and anemia.

Because most of the exposed children do not show symptoms, the only way to identify children at risk is through screening. Lead screening is routinely done during the first years, and it checks the lead level in the blood.

Treatment: Children with high blood lead levels can be treated with medication. But the most important thing is to stop the exposure.

Prevention is the main goal, however. The tools are regular and thorough handwashing and regularly washing the baby's or toddler's pacifiers and toys. Regular cleaning of the household surfaces is necessary in houses built before 1978, when the paint contained lead. The cleaning is particularly important when the house is repainted or remodeled. Be sure that your child is not present when that is happening. Some ceramic vases contain lead. Be sure that your child does not bite or suck on them. Toys made in foreign countries also can contain lead.

Detergents. They can cause vomiting, diarrhea, but if they contain alkali, they can cause burns.

Fluorides. They can cause vomiting, diarrhea, and abdominal pain.

Organic phosphates. They are used in insecticides.
Symptoms are headache, dizziness, diarrhea, sweating, drooling, blurred vision, troubled breathing.
Treatment is atropine.

Many plants, berries, and mushrooms are poisonous. Teach your child not to pick them up and definitely not to eat them.

If there is any suspicion of poisoning, urgent medical attention is necessary.

If significant amount of medication or a poison is ingested, go to the emergency room, or call 911.

Treatment: drinking extra water if the child is conscious, and activated charcoal.

Post-traumatic stress disorder (PTSD)

Children can experience stressful events.

But if a child is strongly affected for a long time, he probable has PTSD.

Symptoms are: reliving the event over and over again, acting hopeless and sad. Sleeping problems are common.

A child with PTSD needs to see a psychologist or a psychiatrist.

Puberty

During puberty, major physical and emotional changes and sexual development take place. There are characteristic changes of the body signaling puberty (see early puberty below). The first signs of puberty in girls is some breast and pubic hair development, and in boys the increased size of the penis and testicles.

Sexual maturation is more closely related to bone maturation than to chronologic age.

Bone age is determined by x-ray of the hand, a good indicator of bone maturation.

A growth spurt is another indication of advancing puberty. It usually occurs between twelve and sixteen years in boys, and between eleven and fourteen years in girls.

In girls, the maximal yearly increase in height usually occurs during the year preceding menarche. In the first year, menstrual periods are often irregular.

Boys often have some *breast enlargement* (*gynecomastia*). It can be on one or both sides, and the breast can be tender. The boy is usually embarrassed about it, and reassurance is in order since it will go away.

Boys and girls who mature later generally are taller than their same-age classmates.

Delayed puberty. Puberty can be delayed as a normal variant (physiologic delay). But there are many other causes as well, like decreased hormonal output of the pituitary gland (panhypopituitarism), head trauma, chronic diseases, tumors, and genetic diseases.

Bone age needs to be checked when a child has delayed puberty.

Laboratory tests include measurements of hormones to find the cause of delayed puberty. Chromosome analysis may be necessary.

If a girl does not have her period by sixteen years of age, *Turner's syndrome* is a possibility.

This condition is caused by a deviation from normal sex chromosomes.

The girl who has this condition is short, she has no sexual development, no menstrual periods. Webbing of the neck is not unusual.

Hormone therapy is available to increase the height and produce some sexual development.

Early puberty (precocious puberty)
A girl has early puberty in general if her sexual development starts before eight years of age, but definitely before seven years if she is white, and six years if she is black.

A boy has early puberty if his sexual development starts before nine years of age.

A child with early puberty may have a growth spurt early on so that he or she becomes taller than others of the same age. However, the final height will be less than that of the others.

There are many causes of early puberty, such as central nervous system disorders or hormone overproduction.

Symptoms of early puberty in girls are enlargement of the breasts, pubic hair, growth spurt, odor in the armpits, early menarche.

Symptoms of early puberty in boys are enlargement of the penis and testicles, pubic hair, growth spurt, odor in the armpits.

The diagnosis is made by history, revealing the age when signs of puberty started. The physical exam shows the height of the child and the physical signs of puberty. X-ray to check the bone age and measurement of hormones is necessary for the diagnosis. Consultation with an endocrinologist is usually necessary.

Treatment is available to slow down the pubertal development.

Rash

Heat rash (prickly heat)

Heat rash is caused by sweating from hot, humid weather, strenuous exercise, and high fever.

Tiny red bumps develop, mostly on the chest, back, and abdomen.

Have your child in a cooler place, and keep him or her in light, loose cloth.

If your child has blisters on the skin, scalp, often in the mouth, and fever, *chickenpox* is a good possibility. After a few days, red bumps, blisters, and scabs can be seen at the same time.

If your child has high fever, watery pink eye, cough, runny nose for few days and then red spots appear all over the skin, there is a suspicion of *measles*.

If your child has fever, pink eye, a rash with small pink spots, and small lumps (enlarged lymph nodes) at the back of the head, *German measles*-rubella is likely.

If your child has high fever for three days without any other symptoms and feels okay, then a pink rash develops but there is no more fever, your baby or child probably has *roseola*.

If your child has a red face and a fine pink lacelike rash on the arms and legs but there is no fever, he or she probably has *fifth disease*. This rash can stay on for weeks.

Many diseases caused by other viruses can have rash as well.

If your child has fever, sore throat, a very red or white tongue, and a fine reddish rough rash at the lower part of the abdomen and the inner side of the arms, the likely diagnosis is *scarlet fever*.

(For all the above diseases, see infectious diseases of childhood.)

All of these diseases are contagious.

Rocky Mountain spotted fever. (See fever.)

(See also the chapter about itchy skin.)

If your child has a rash, visit the doctor. On the telephone, let the office know if you suspect a contagious disease so as not to infect others.

Sepsis

Sepsis is a serious condition caused by germs present in the bloodstream and the body's response to the infection.

Symptoms are high fever, chills, vomiting, diarrhea, headache, weakness.

Sepsis can lead to the injury of different organs.

Diagnosis is made by history, physical exam, and blood tests (CBC, blood culture).

Treatment:

- Intravenous (through the vein) antibiotics
- Intravenous fluids
- Corticosteroids
- Oxygen if needed

Sexually transmitted diseases (STD), also called venereal diseases

If an adolescent girl or boy has sores, warts, or blisters at the genital area, or a discharge from the vagina or penis, there is a suspicion of STD. Painful urination can also be a symptom. If any of these symptoms are present, a visit to the doctor is imperative.

Prevention is most important. The use of a condom all the time gives a high percentage of protection against sexually transmitted diseases and pregnancy.

If a girl is sexually active, a visit with a gynecologist is recommended.

Since sexually transmitted diseases not always show symptoms, screening tests are needed to make the diagnosis. Some sexually transmitted diseases can be dangerous if not treated. But if they are treated in time, they can be cured. There is a recommendation for young people to get tested for HIV and other sexually transmitted diseases.

Common sexually transmitted diseases are syphilis, chlamydia, gonorrhea, herpes, trichomoniasis, human immunodeficiency virus (HIV), and warts (condyloma acuminata).

Syphilis

Syphilis is a severe chronic systemic disease.
It is caused by bacteria called *Treponema pallidum*.
The disease has different phases: primary, secondary, tertiary.

Primary syphilis. This starts with a bump that becomes a painless sore (ulcer) on the genital, called chancre. Local lymph nodes are enlarged. The ulcer heals with a scar.

If the adolescent is untreated, the next phase will develop.

Secondary syphilis. A rash develops and covers the whole body. Other symptoms are low-grade fever, malaise, headache, weight loss, and muscle and joint pain. The eyes, kidneys, and liver can be involved. Meningitis can also be present.

Tertiary syphilis. Heart and neurologic problems can show up, as well as lumps (gumma) in the skin and muscles.

Syphilis can be transmitted from the mother to the newborn. The symptoms often develop only a few weeks or months after birth. An early sign is a stuffy nose. The disease can affect multiple organs. Rash, enlargement of the liver, spleen, and lymph nodes are common.

Bone, kidney, eye involvement, and central nervous system abnormalities can be present.

Diagnosis is made by blood tests. A screening test of the mother for syphilis is included in prenatal care.

Therapy is penicillin (see infections that can harm the fetus).

Chlamydia and gonorrhea

Chlamydia is caused by bacteria called *Chlamydia trachomatis*, and gonorrhea is caused by a bacteria called *gonococcus*.

Chlamydia and gonorrhea in a girl can cause *pelvic inflammatory disease (PID)*.

Symptoms are lower abdominal pain and tenderness. Pain also can be elicited by gynecologic exam. There is often fever, vomiting, and vaginal discharge.

The diagnosis is made by the symptoms, physical findings, and laboratory tests.

Pelvic inflammatory disease can cause sterility.

Therapy is antibiotics.

Genital herpes

Herpes is caused by the herpes virus. The presentation of genital herpes is small painful bumps, blisters or sores (ulcers) at the genital area. These lesions often recur.

Mothers can transmit the infection to their newborn, causing severe infection. Blisters can be seen on the skin, and the disease can involve the brain, eyes, and liver.

Testing can be done from the fluid in the blisters.

Treatment is antiviral therapy, like acyclovir. (See infections that can harm the fetus.)

Trichomoniasis

It is caused by a parasite that has only one cell (protozoa). The symptom of a trichomonas infection is genital discharge.

Diagnosis is made by laboratory test from the discharge.

Therapy is a drug called metronidazole.

Human immunodeficiency virus infection (HIV/AIDS)

The advanced stage of HIV infection is called *acquired immunodeficiency syndrome (AIDS)*.

HIV infection disables the body's immune system to fight infections. Bacterial, viral, and fungal infections can develop, as well as tumors.

Enlarged lymph nodes, spleen, and liver are often present.

The disease can be transmitted from the mother to her newborn.

Diagnosis is made by blood test.

Treatment is antiretroviral therapy (medications). These drugs are also used to treat pregnant women to prevent transmission to the newborn (see infections that can harm the fetus).

Genital warts (condyloma acuminata)

It is caused by the *human papilloma virus* (*HPV*).

The papilloma virus can cause genital cancer; therefore, HPV shot is now part of the immunization schedule.

In case of any sexually transmitted disease, it is important to treat the partner.

Early diagnosis and treatment of these diseases is extremely important to prevent serious complications.

Sickness all the time—the child who is always sick (immunodeficiency)

If a child is frequently sick with significant illnesses or gets unusual infections, there is a suspicion that the child's immune system does not work right. The child might have a condition called *immunodeficiency.*

Important questions:

- How often does the child get sick?
- How long does the illness last?
- What kind of infections does the child have?
- How severe are the infections?
- Has he been hospitalized?
- Has he fully recovered?
- How much time passes between infections?
- Has the child had any unusual infection?
- Is anybody sick at home?
- Is there anybody in the family who is always sick?
- Does anybody in the family have immunodeficiency?
- How many days did he miss school?

Children can have frequent colds (viral infections) in general. Babies are more susceptible to infections. The ability to fight infections improves with age.

Children attending day care are exposed to more germs and viruses than those who are at home.

The immunodeficiency can be cellular (severe combined immunodeficiency), meaning that the problem is with the cells belonging to the immune system that fights infections, or humoral (common variable immunodeficiency), when the gamma globulin is absent or diminished (see below).

Children with immunodeficiency have increased susceptibility to bacterial, viral, and fungal infections. Chronic ear and sinus infections are frequent. They can have recurrent pneumonia, meningitis, skin infections, bone infections, etc.

If a baby or a child has white spots on the tongue and inside the mouth, oral thrush (yeast infection-monilia), after being treated over a month, immunodeficiency is suspected.

The immunodeficiency can be transient or permanent. Most of the permanent immunodeficiencies are inherited.

Transient immunodeficiencies are the following:

Transient hypogammaglobulinemia. This is a condition when the infant has low immunoglobulin level in the blood over six months of age. Most children will grow it out between the ages of two and five.

Transient acquired immunodeficiency. This means that the immune system is weakened. It can be caused by certain medications (chemotherapy for cancer) and viruses.

Primary immunodeficiencies. These are permanent. They are usually inherited. The diagnosis is made by the history, physical exam, and laboratory tests.

There are many types of primary immunodeficiencies.

Common variable immunodeficiency (CVID). This is an inherited disease.

Children with this genetic disorder have low levels of antibodies to fight infections (antibodies are proteins made by the immune system to fight specific infections).

Severe combined immunodeficiency. This means that the child is not able to produce immune cells. This is a rare genetic disorder.

Agammaglobulinemia. This is also a genetic disorder. The child cannot make antibodies to fight infections.

Treatment of immunodeficiencies:

- Immunoglobulin replacement.
- Antibiotics to fight infections.
- Good hygiene.
- Avoid crowds and people who have cold or other infections.
- Bone marrow transplant in case of severe combined immunodeficiency.

Children with immunodeficiencies cannot receive live vaccines. Also immunocompromised children, like those who have HIV, cancer, organ transplant, or receiving chemotherapy or radiation, cannot have these vaccines.

Live vaccines are rotavirus, live polio vaccine (OPV), MMR (measles, mumps, rubella), Varivax (chickenpox), MMRV (measles, mumps, rubella, chickenpox) (see immunizations).

Pediatric immunologist or allergist/immunologist and pediatric infectious disease specialists are usually involved in the care of children with immunodeficiencies.

Sinus infection (sinusitis)

The nasal discharge is usually clear when a child has an upper respiratory infection. It can turn to yellow, then green, but it becomes clear again. It usually resolves after seven to ten days.

However, if the nasal discharge lasts longer than ten to fourteen days, and the mucus remains green, sinus infection (sinusitis) is suspected. That means that a bacterial infection developed.

The bacteria causing the infection is most commonly *Pneumococcus, Streptococcus*, and *Haemophilus influenzae*. Allergies can contribute to the development of a sinus infection.

Symptoms are often thick green nasal mucus, pain, tenderness, and feeling fullness over the sinuses. The location of the pain is the forehead and the face. The pain increases when the child bends over. Fever, malaise, and cough often accompany the disease.

The most common sinus infection is *maxillary sinusitis*. The maxillary sinuses are located on the face under the eye sockets (orbits).

The frontal sinus is located at the eyebrows, and the infection of the frontal sinus (*frontal sinusitis*) often causes headache. The ethmoid sinus is located behind the nose. The infection of the ethmoid sinus (*ethmoiditis*) can cause swelling around the eye, indicating *periorbital cellulitis* (see cellulitis in the chapter "Skin Infections").

Sometimes an x-ray can help to establish the diagnosis of a sinus infection. Limited CT scan, and rarely MRI, can be used as well.

Complications can occur, like infection of the membranes around the brain (meningitis) or infection of the bone (osteomyelitis).

Treatment is antibiotic.

Often an ENT (ear, nose, and throat) doctor is participating in the care of the child.

Skin infections

Skin infections are common and may be caused by bacteria, viruses, or fungi. The clinical picture of a bacterial infection depends on the depth of the skin involved.

The most common germs causing skin infections are *Streptococcus pyogenes* and *Staphylococcus aureus*.

Many times the infection starts with a bug bite, scratch, or a little cut.

Common bacterial infections:

- impetigo (most superficial)
- boils (furuncles)
- cellulitis
- abscess

Common viral infections:

- chickenpox (see infectious diseases)
- herpes infections (see viral infections)

Common fungal infections:

- athlete's foot (see athlete's foot)
- yeast-monilial diaper rash (see itchy skin)

Impetigo. Impetigo is contagious.

The child can have blisters on the skin, or sores with crusts. They can develop anywhere in the body. The cause of impetigo is most often group A *Streptococcus* (also causing strep throat) and *Staphylococcus aureus.*

Since impetigo is a bacterial disease, the child needs to see the doctor for proper medications.

The treatment can be antibiotic ointment if only very few small lesions are present. Otherwise the treatment is antibiotic by mouth.

Sometimes inflammation of the kidneys (glomerulonephritis) develops. Proper antibiotic treatment decreases the occurrence of kidney disease.

Boils (furuncles). Boils are bacterial infections. The bacteria *Staphylococcus aureus* is often the cause. They can develop anywhere in the body, but more often on the face, nose, neck, and buttocks. They can start from a cut, bite, or a hair follicle.

They are painful, tender red bumps. When the middle of the bump gets soft and yellowish, containing pus, it often bursts, and the pus comes out. It can resolve that way.

A *cluster of boils is called carbuncle.* Lymph nodes often get enlarged in the area where the boil is present.

Therapy: For pimples and small boils, antibiotic ointments can be tried. Sterile gauze should cover it. If the boil is large or growing, oral antibiotics are needed. See the doctor. If the large boil gets soft, it needs to be opened (incision and drainage).

Cellulitis. Cellulitis is a skin infection that affects the deeper layer of the skin. It can start with a bite, scratch, or cut. It can be anywhere on the skin, but it is more common on the arms and legs. The germs causing cellulitis most commonly are *Staphylococcus aureus* and *Streptococcus pyogenes.*

The signs of cellulites are redness, swelling, tenderness, and warmth in the area. Fever and enlargement of lymph nodes in the area are common.

Therapy is antibiotics.

Cellulitis around the eye is called *periorbital cellulitis.*

In case of periorbital cellulitis, there is swelling and redness of the eyelid and around the eye. It often originates in sinus infection (ethmoid sinusitis). The germs causing it are usually *Staphylococcus, Streptococcus* and *Haemophilus influenzae* (H. flu).

If the child cannot move his or her eye, that means that the eye is involved too (*orbital cellulitis*). That is an even more severe condition. If there is suspicion of periorbital or orbital cellulitis, go to the emergency room.

Treatment of periorbital and orbital cellulitis requires hospitalization and aggressive antibiotic therapy, often with the antibiotic injected into the vein (intravenous, or IV therapy). In case of orbital cellulitis, an eye doctor (ophthalmologist) is involved in the child's care.

Skin abscess. Skin abscess develops in the deeper area of the skin. *Staphylococcus* and *Streptococcus* are the most common bacteria causing it. It can develop anywhere on the skin.

Abscess starts as a firm, tender red nodule. Later it gets soft.

Treatment is surgery. The abscess needs to be opened or removed. Antibiotics are also often used.

The abscess is often packed with sterile gauze that is removed later to bring out the pus from the abscess.

With the exception of small boils, all of these conditions need medical attention.

Molluscum contagiosum. Molluscum contagiosum is a viral infection causing skin lesions. These are small, firm, painless flesh-colored bumps with indentation in the middle. The bumps have a pearly appearance.

They can spread in the following ways:

- From person to person with skin-to-skin contact.
- Contaminated objects.
- Sexual contact.
- Scratching or rubbing the skin can spread the lesions to other parts of the skin.

These bumps may appear anywhere on the skin.

Molluscum contagiosum is self-limited, so treatment is usually not necessary. It disappears in a few months or a year. Removal is possible.

Paronychia. Paronychia is an infection of the skin that surrounds a fingernail or a toenail.

It usually starts with cutting the nail and cutting into the skin. The infection then is caused by a bacteria. The area gets red, warm, swollen, painful, and tender to the touch. Maybe pus can be seen as well. If your child has these symptoms, see the doctor.

Treatment is soaking the finger or toe in Betadine (iodine). Dilute the Betadine with water—three-fourths of betadine, one-fourths of water. Soak it for ten minutes, three times a day, then remove the Betadine with alcohol or water.

Sometimes antibiotic treatment is necessary, but if pus accumulates, it might need to be drained.

There is a chronic form of paronychia as well, caused by a fungus called *Candida.* In that case, the symptoms develop slowly.

Treatment is antifungal ointment.

Treatment of paronychia:

- Soaking with Betadine
- Antibiotics if needed
- Surgery if necessary

Prevention:

- Keep the hands and feet clean and dry.
- Be careful when cutting the nails. Do not cut it too short.
- Avoid nail biting. You want to praise your child when he does not bite his nails. Also, you can use positive reinforcement. You tell your child if he does not bite his nails for a certain period of time, like an hour or two, you give a star or a small sticker, and put it in a notebook. After awarding

a certain number of stars or stickers, the child will get a small present. The task should not be too easy or too hard.
• Avoid sucking on a finger.

Sleep, sleep problems

Newborn babies usually sleep during the day and are up at night. They often cry at night, particularly if they are hungry or wet. The first few weeks are hard for mothers because they do not get enough sleep. It is important to sleep during the day, between feedings.

But even when you are tired, pick up the baby for feedings, and do not prop the bottle, because that can be dangerous.

Even when your baby is older and able to hold the bottle, do not let him or her fall asleep with it. It can cause choking and tooth decay, the so-called "nursing bottle teeth."

The damage of the teeth, the cavities, can be so large and deep that the tops of the teeth are missing.

Premature babies may need night feedings. Often babies do not want to give up their night feedings. If that is the case, cut one night feeding at a time until the night feedings are stopped. First you want to get rid of the feeding in the middle of the night. When your baby sleeps over that feeding, you can work on the others. You can give your baby one or two ounces of water instead of the feeding. The water should be boiled first, and one teaspoon of sugar added to four ounces of water. Do not give more than two ounces of water per day. You also want to comfort your baby if he or she cries when you make the change. After several days (it varies how long), your baby will get used to the new routine.

Keep your baby in your room for at least the first six months of life, preferably for the first year. Your baby should sleep on his or her back on a firm mattress in the crib. Keep soft objects, pillows, stuffed animals out of the crib to prevent suffocation or sudden infant death syndrome (SIDS) or sudden unexpected infant death (SUID).

Do not use inclined sleepers, in-bed sleepers, soft padding, crib bumpers for the same safety reasons.

Do not sleep in the same bed with your baby because you can injure him or her by rolling over the baby. Products that are for bed-sharing with parents are not safe either.

It is important to check on your baby always when crying to be sure that there is nothing wrong with him or her. You want to see that your baby's diaper is not wet or soiled and that he or she has no fever, vomiting, or diarrhea. You want to be sure that his color and breathing is okay, and that he or she responds as usual. Be sure that the baby does not have a rash, a bite, or redness or swelling anywhere on the body, and there is no hair around his finger. Teething and ear infection are common causes of crying at night. Also, colic is a common cause of stomachache during the first two to three months. Pick up your baby and smile. That often stops the crying and then you know your baby is okay. If the baby screams for hours and nothing stops it, medical attention is needed. Go to the emergency room.

Everybody needs different amounts of sleep. Babies and children need more sleep than adults. Newborn babies can sleep sixteen to twenty hours a day. Babies usually sleep twelve hours at night and take two naps. Toddlers sleep about the same hours but take only one nap.

After five years of age, children require about ten hours of sleep. Adolescents should sleep at least eight hours (they often do not), but they like to get up late whenever they can.

Sleeping problems are not uncommon in childhood and are even more common among adolescents.

Adolescents often watch exciting TV shows and play video games for a long time before going to bed. It is no surprise that they cannot fall asleep, being too wired. They are sleepy in the morning, so their school performance is often affected. They also can be irritated because of the lack of sleep.

Children can refuse to go to bed and want to stay up to continue their activities. They may want to see what the adults are doing or talking about. They also can be scared of darkness, strange shadows, noises, or being separated from their parents. Leaving the door open and a night-light can help. Many times they also want to watch TV, play video games, and use their iPhones. No media should be in the bedroom.

Do not let him do vigorous exercise within four hours before bedtime.

Avoid coffee, Coke, and tea.

Your child should not take a daytime nap, or only a very short one.

Nightmares are not uncommon. A bad dream wakes the child up, and he or she goes to the bed of the parents or a sibling. Parental reassurance and a night-light are needed.

In case of *night terror*, the child wakes up frightened and confused. There is sweating, fast breathing, and pulse. The child does not wake up fully even when the parents try to wake him or her.

The child has no recollection of the event in the morning.

Obstructive sleep apnea. The child stops breathing for a few seconds, then takes a deep breath and breathes normally. It can happen several times a night, and the child is sleepy in the morning because of the disturbed sleep. It usually happens when the tonsils and adenoids are enlarged, and the child is often obese. Loud snoring is characteristic.

Sleep apnea needs medical attention. See the doctor. Often sleep study (polysomnography) and an ENT (ear, nose, and throat doctor) consult is necessary.

Insomnia. Insomnia means that the child has a problem falling asleep or staying asleep at night.

It can be caused by stress but can also be a sign of depression.

It is important to develop a healthy nighttime routine. Have a quiet family dinner. A little walk is good too, but heavy exercise is not. Avoid your child watching exciting TV shows or playing video games close to bedtime. Reading a book that is not too exciting before bedtime can be also useful. Your child should not drink much close to bedtime, and be sure that he or she goes to the bathroom before going to bed. As I mentioned before, be sure that your child does not drink coffee, tea, or coke in the evening. (They do not suppose to drink those anyway). If the insomnia does not improve, see the doctor.

Sleep walking (somnambulism). The child gets up and walks while sleeping.

The only important thing is to prevent injuries.

Lock the windows and doors. Remove potentially dangerous objects, and block the staircase for the night.

The child has no memory of what happened.

They usually outgrow this condition.

Narcolepsy. Narcolepsy is a sleep disorder. The child has an uncontrollable sleepiness and frequently falls asleep.

If the child has severe sleeping problems, see the doctor.

Also a sleep doctor can be consulted. Sometimes an overnight sleep study (polysomnography) is necessary.

Sneezing

Occasional sneezing is common.

Influenza and common colds (URI) are viral infections and cause sneezing and coughing. Cover your nose and mouth when sneezing.

Sunshine often provokes sneezing.

But if your child has several sneezes in a row (sneezing spell), particularly if he also rubs his nose, then allergy, hay fever, is likely. In that case, it is advisable to see the doctor.

Snoring

If a child regularly snores, that usually indicates that his sleep is disturbed. That also means that he is tired the next day.

Frequent causes of snoring are enlarged adenoids and tonsils.

If the child stops breathing for a few seconds, then gasping for air, he probably has obstructive sleep apnea secondary to enlarged adenoids and tonsils.

Another cause is nasal blockage from allergies (allergic rhinitis) or a deviated nasal septum.

If your child has significant snoring regularly, see the doctor.

Sleep study can help to make the diagnosis. Often a referral to an ear, nose, and throat specialist is necessary.

Soiling of the pants (encopresis)

Encopresis is the soiling of the pants after four years of age. It can happen when the child has never been fully trained, or it can recur.

Soiling of the pants is often caused by constipation (see constipation). The rectum is full with hard stool, and some softer stool overflows. If the constipation causes crack at the rectum, that leads to the withholding of more stool because of the pain when having a bowel movement.

Some children have problems holding the stool and the urine up to a certain age. But if the child has no physical or mental problem, it should be resolved spontaneously.

Emotional problems can also cause soiling of the pants. It can start with too early or harsh toilet training. Later, scolding and discipline about accidents can add to the problem.

Treatment:

You want to stop the constipation. It is important for your child to have regular, normal stools. (See constipation.)

Reassure your child of your support and of the fact that the problem will go away eventually.

You want to explain to him or her that the maturation of the body happens gradually. For some children it happens sooner, while for others it takes longer.

Cooperation of the child is very important. It is important that you do not scold or discipline your child for accidents and show no frustration or talk about inconvenience. Praise your child for any improvement, and you may give little presents for success. (See bed-wetting.) If the cause is emotional problem, a psychologist may need to be involved in the child's care.

Sore throat (pharyngitis)

Sore throats are caused by bacteria and viruses. The most important bacteria is *group A Streptococcus* (GAS), that causes strep throat and tonsillitis. Scarlet fever is another manifestation (see rash).

Sore throat is often accompanied with other symptoms: fever, headache, stomachache, and vomiting. Children often refuse to eat or drink because of the pain when they swallow. In extreme cases, it can lead to dehydration. Enlargement of lymph nodes on the neck is also common.

Strep throat can be detected by physical exam and confirmed by throat culture. There is also a rapid strep test. If it is positive, it confirms the diagnosis of strep throat. However, if it is negative, that does not rule it out. Therefore, if the rapid test is negative, a regular throat culture is done.

Parents often say, "The child just has a sore throat." "He got a fever reducer, and the fever stopped after two days." "We thought everything was okay." But the problem is, that after an untreated or not sufficiently treated strep throat, the child can develop a secondary disease, affecting the heart— acute rheumatic fever (see joint pain with systemic diseases)—or kidney—acute poststreptococcal glomerulonephritis (see blood in the urine). Sydenham's chorea can develop as well (see jerking and strange movements).

Therefore, sore throats always need medical attention.

The treatment of strep throat is antibiotic therapy. The drug of choice is penicillin (often amoxicillin is used). Sometimes there is a need for another antibiotic, like cephalosporin. Always give the antibiotic regularly, and finish the full course of ten days even if the child feels better after a few days. It is very important not to skip even one dose. You want to give your child plenty of fluids and acetaminophen or ibuprofen for fever or pain. Lozenges, honey, and candy also can help.

The tonsils and adenoids are small masses of tissues. Both are part of the immune system.

Tonsils are located in the throat on both sides, while the adenoids are in the nasopharynx, behind the nose. During a physical exam, the doctor can see the tonsils with the naked eyes, but not the adenoids.

The tonsils often get infected (*tonsillitis*), mostly with the germ group A *Streptococcus*, as in strep throat. The tonsils are enlarged, red, and often white spots can be seen.

Chronic tonsillitis means that the child has persistent or recurrent sore throats.

The tonsils are enlarged and scarred.

The treatment of tonsillitis is antibiotic, used the same way as in strep throat. If tonsillitis frequently recurs, the removal of the tonsils can be necessary. The name of the surgery is tonsillectomy.

Scarlet fever is also caused by group A *Streptococcus*.

The incubation period is two to five days.

The symptoms are sore throat, fever, and often vomiting and a rash. The rash is small red spots, often confluent and mostly located on the chest, abdomen, and the inner surface of the arms. The rash is rough to the touch. The tongue can be red with red bumps (red strawberry tongue), or coated, white with red bumps (white strawberry tongue). Complications and treatment are the same like in case of strep throat (see infectious diseases of childhood).

If the child with tonsillitis is not getting better on antibiotic treatment, there is a suspicion that he or she has mononucleosis. A child can also have mononucleosis and strep throat together (see mononucleosis).

Infection of the tonsils can spread to the surrounding tissues, and abscess formation can be the consequence (*peritonsillar abscess*). It usually occurs on one side.

Symptoms are severe sore throat and high fever. If the infection is severe, drooling and problems swallowing (dysphagia) can develop.

Treatment:

- Hospital admission is often necessary.
- Antibiotics (usually IV)

- Consult with an otolaryngologist (ENT)
- Surgery is usually necessary to open and drain the abscess.

An abscess can also develop behind the pharynx (back of the throat) (*retropharyngeal abscess*).

Symptoms are fever, irritability, and problems swallowing and breathing.

Treatment:

- Hospital admission
- Antibiotics (IV)
- Consult with an otolaryngologist
- Surgery

Adenoiditis. Adenoiditis often occurs with tonsillitis.

Acute adenoiditis can cause fever, vomiting, headache, but the child also has nasal congestion, snoring, and difficulty sleeping.

If the child has chronic adenoid infections, the adenoids get enlarged.

The child cannot breathe through the nose, so he or she will breathe through the mouth (mouth breathing). Symptoms are muffled, nasal voice and snoring at night.

Enlarged adenoids can cause chronic ear infection by blocking the Eustachian tube. The Eustachian tube connects the middle ear with the nose.

Enlarged adenoids can cause the breathing to stop for a few seconds—*obstructive sleep apnea* (see sleep and sleep disorders).

If the tonsils and adenoids are extremely large, they can block the airway, and the child has a problem breathing, particularly at night. If this problem is severe, urgent medical attention is needed. Call 911. In the meantime, keep the child in a sitting position.

If the problem breathing is present in a lesser degree but for a long time, and the child does not get sufficient amounts of oxygen, the heart can be affected (*cor pulmonale*).

Tonsils are usually larger during childhood and shrink in the teenage years. The tonsils do not need to be removed just because they are enlarged if they cause no symptoms.

However, if the tonsils and adenoids are so enlarged that they cause disturbed sleep, heart problems, trouble swallowing and/or breathing, the removal of the tonsils and adenoids is indicated (tonsillectomy and adenoidectomy). An ear, nose, and throat (ENT) doctor will do the surgery.

Splinters

It is not uncommon for children to get splinters in their fingers or soles.

Splinters can hurt when pressure is applied or the child walks on it.

Remove the splinter as soon as possible because it is easier to pull it out, and it is less likely to get infected.

Clean your hands first and then clean the area with the splinter with soap and water. Sterilize a needle and tweezers with alcohol, keeping the tips in alcohol for ten minutes.

If the end of the splinter is still poking out of the skin, gently remove it with a tweezer.

If the splinter is under the skin, gently scrape the skin with the sterile needle until you can grab it with the tweezer. Be sure there is no part of the splinter left inside. Put alcohol, peroxide, or Betadine to the area, and use an antibiotic ointment like Neosporin. Finally, cover it with a sterile bandage.

But your child needs medical attention in the following circumstances:

- If the wound is bleeding much
- If the splinter is deep in the tissues
- If you cannot remove the splinter easily
- If the area seems to be infected, being red, swollen, and tender
- If the splinter is close to the eye
- If it is under the fingernail
- If the splinter is embedded for a while
- If your child is not up-to-date on tetanus immunizations, or more than five years passed since he received the last tetanus shot

Sprains

A sprain is the stretching or tearing of the ligament. Ligaments connect two bones together in a joint.

The most common sprain is in the ankle.

Symptoms are pain, swelling, bruising, and limited mobility. Sometimes a "pop" can be heard.

If the sprain is severe, the ligament can be torn.

The diagnosis is made by history, physical exam, but often an x-ray and MRI is needed.

The initial treatment is RICE: rest, ice, compression, elevation (see muscle strain).

Tylenol or ibuprofen can help the pain.

Your child can use crutches if necessary.

Orthopedic specialists treat severe sprains.

A splint or cast can be used to immobilize the area.

Surgery can be necessary.

It is important that your child stay away from sports until the doctor recommends it.

Prevention is stretching and strengthening exercising before playing sports.

Stature—short stature and tall stature

Short stature. The height of a child is mostly determined by the height of the parents; therefore, family history is very important. Nutrition is important as well.

A child who has short stature is below the 3 percentile on the growth chart (see growth and development/growth charts).

The height of premature babies is lower than that of term babies in the first two years. Babies who were small for gestational age (SGA) are also shorter. That can be caused by insufficient nutrition through the placenta. The placenta itself can be damaged. They may show catch-up growth and reach their height potential. But SGA also can be caused by diseases during pregnancy, alcohol abuse (fetal alcohol syndrome), and heavy smoking of the mother.

Naturally a child can be short if his parents and relatives are short.

During childhood, the cause of short stature can be inadequate nutrition and chronic disease affecting any organs in the body, like the heart, kidney, and liver. Genetic and endocrine disorders also can cause short stature. Early puberty can also cause short stature because the growth plates close earlier. However, children with early puberty will have a growth spurt earlier, so the child will be taller than his or her peers at a given time, even as the adult height will be less than theirs.

On the other hand, if puberty is delayed, the child will be short throughout the childhood, but if everything is okay otherwise, the adult height will be normal.

The endocrine disorders leading to short stature are insufficient secretion of the thyroid hormone or the growth hormone.

Insufficient secretion of the thyroid hormone

That is caused by *deficient activity of the thyroid gland—hypothyroidism.* The newborn screening tests include screening for this condition because it can be congenital.

Therefore, the second newborn screening test that is done at two weeks of age is important (the first test is done in the newborn nursery). If the laboratory tests confirm the diagnosis, the baby needs treatment with thyroid hormone. That is very important, because without appropriate and early treatment, the baby may be mentally deficient. But hypothyroidism can develop later on as well. Infection, or most often an autoimmune disease, called *Hashimoto's thyroiditis*, is the cause. In this case, the body acts against the body's own tissue. The symptoms are dry skin, coarse hair, constipation, often enlarged thyroid gland. Also, there is an increase in weight, a decrease in height, and a delayed puberty. Thyroid hormone therapy is necessary.

Short stature in girls can also be caused by a genetic disorder called Turner syndrome. In that case, there is no sexual development by age sixteen. (See menstrual period (menstrual cycle), menstrual problems).

Insufficient secretion of growth hormone

If a child has *growth hormone deficiency*, hypopituitarism, he or she is short for the age. The child looks younger than his or her age. Puberty can be delayed.

Diagnosis is made by laboratory tests.

Treatment is growth hormone therapy.

Tall stature. A child with tall stature is over 97 percent on the growth chart.

A child can be very tall if his or her parents and relatives are very tall. Family history is important.

But tall stature can develop if the pituitary gland produces an excessive amount of growth hormone.

The condition is called *gigantism* and requires medical investigation for the cause because it can be caused by a tumor of the pituitary gland.

If a child is very tall, has very long arms, fingers, and toes, there is a suspicion that he or she might have *Marfan syndrome*. A child with Marfan syndrome also has lax joints, eye problems, and could have heart problems. The child needs to be closely watched because curvature of the spine (scoliosis) can develop.

Stomachache (abdominal pain)

Stomachache is a very common complaint. It can be mild or severe.

It can be caused by a benign or a severe condition.

Important questions:

- Is this the first time he or she has this kind of pain? If the answer is no, how often has the pain recurred?
- When did the pain start?
- Is the pain severe? Ask your child to rate it from one to ten (one is the mildest, ten is the strongest pain).
- Does the pain radiate anywhere? If the answer is yes, where does it radiate?
- How is the child's appetite?
- Is the pain related to eating? If the answer is yes, is the pain before or after eating, and for how long?
- What makes the pain better or worse?
- Has the child had any vomiting, diarrhea, fever, or complaints with urination?
- How often does he or she urinate and have a bowel movement? When was the last urination and bowel movement?
- How do the stools look, and are they normal or hard?

The child's age is important. A young baby can have stomachache caused by gas, *colic* (see at home with your new baby). Also, milk allergy can cause abdominal pain. If a baby has a stomachache, the parents can only guess it. The baby is fussy, crying, kicking, does not want to eat, and does not act right.

If a young baby has abdominal pain with severe constipation and vomiting and distended abdomen, Hirschsprung disease is a possibility. In that case, there is a lack of nerve cells in the large bowel (see constipation). If Hirschsprung disease is suspected, medical attention is needed. But if the abdomen is swollen and the baby vomits, go to the emergency room.

Acute abdominal pain

Abdominal pain and vomiting. If a child has a stomachache and vomits once or twice, and after that he or she feels fine, has no other complaints or symptoms, the cause can be overeating or having something that did not agree with the child's stomach. In this case, the child feels much better after vomiting. He or she only needs to be on a diet for a day or so. The diet is clear liquids and the so-called BRAT diet (banana, rice, applesauce, and toast). Give the clear liquids cold, and start it slowly. If the child keeps the fluids down, you can start a piece of toast and applesauce in after about eight hours.

After that, gradually go back to regular diet. Fried, heavy foods and milk and dairy products should be the last ones reintroduced.

However, if the child vomits two to three times and the pain continues, urgent medical attention is necessary.

Continuous vomiting can lead to dehydration. If the child has no urine for eight to nine hours, that indicates dehydration. Go to the emergency room. If the child has severe abdominal pain, cries, holds his or her stomach, bends over, and vomits, go to the emergency room, or call 911.

Abdominal pain and vomiting can be symptoms of severe conditions, like bowel obstruction and bowel perforation (acute abdomen).

Acute abdomen

Acute abdomen is a serious condition that starts with sudden, severe abdominal pain.

Other symptoms are vomiting, abdominal tenderness, and involuntary guarding (the abdominal wall is tense when the doctor checks his abdomen). The abdomen is rigid.

Acute abdomen is an emergency. If your child has sudden, severe abdominal pain and vomiting, go to the emergency room, or call 911.

A surgeon is generally consulted.

A sonogram or CT scan of the abdomen helps to make the diagnosis.

Treatment is often surgery.

Bowel obstruction. This occurs when the small or large bowel is blocked, preventing the passage of foods.

There are many causes of bowel obstruction:

- Twisted intestine (volvulus)
- Trapped hernia, incarcerated hernia (see hernia)
- Scar tissues (adhesions) from previous surgery
- Intussusception (see vomiting)
- Crohn's disease (see stomachache)
- Bulging pouches (diverticulums)
- Impacted stool

Bleeding. This is an injury of an organ. If a girl has vaginal bleeding not related to her period, it can be ectopic pregnancy. Go to the emergency room, or call 911 (see below).

Bowel perforation. This means that a hole forms in the small or large intestine. The contents of the bowel leak into the abdominal cavity, and that can lead to a severe infection and inflammation of the peritoneum, called *peritonitis.* The peritoneum is a membrane that lines the inner abdominal wall and covers the organs of the abdomen.

Some causes of bowel perforation are the following:

- Blunt trauma
- Foreign bodies, particularly small batteries
- Bowel obstruction
- Appendicitis
- Meckel diverticulum (see below)
- Peptic ulcer disease

Symptoms are severe abdominal pain, vomiting, and fever. Shock can develop as well. (see change in consciousness, fast breathing, cold sweat).

X-rays, CT scan, and endoscopy (see tests and procedures, surgeries) are the tests helping to make the diagnosis.

Treatment is surgery.

Abdominal pain, vomiting, fever. Babies can have any illness with fever and vomiting. Ear infection is a good example.

Common diseases that can cause abdominal pain, vomiting, and fever are strep throat, pneumonia, and viral diseases like hepatitis.

However, these symptoms also can indicate severe conditions, like *appendicitis.* In that case, the pain is usually located at the right lower side of the abdomen. But the pain sometimes is localized in the middle of the abdomen.

Urgent medical attention is needed. Go to the emergency room. Do not wait, because if the appendix perforates, severe infection can develop in the abdomen (peritonitis).

Pancreatitis. Pancreatitis is an inflammation of the pancreas, a large gland located behind the stomach. The pancreas produces digestive enzymes and the hormones insulin and glucagon. These hormones regulate the blood sugar.

Symptoms: Abdominal pain is present in both acute and chronic pancreatitis. The pain is in the upper abdomen and may radiate to the back.

In acute pancreatitis, the symptoms are abdominal pain, fever, nausea, vomiting, and swollen and tender abdomen.

In chronic pancreatitis, there is diarrhea and weight loss.

If the pancreas is inflamed, the enzymes amylase and lipase are elevated.

Diagnosis is made by blood tests showing elevated enzymes (amylase and lipase), ultrasound, CT scan, or MRI.

Treatment depends on severity.

Abdominal pain, vomiting and diarrhea. Abdominal pain, vomiting, and diarrhea is most commonly seen in *gastroenteritis*, which is the inflammation of the stomach and bowels. It can be caused by bacterial or viral infections. Some parasites can cause these symptoms as well. Fever is also often present. It can lead to dehydration. Take your child to the doctor.

Treatment depends on the cause. But to keep a diet is always necessary. Start with cold, clear liquids slowly, then follow the BRAT diet (see diarrhea).

Intussusception. This is a bowel obstruction caused by a part of the intestine sliding into another part of the intestine.

Usually infants and young children have it.

Symptoms: episodes of severe abdominal pain, vomiting, stool mixed with blood and mucus, and the stool looks like currant jelly.

The child can get dehydrated (see dehydration).

Intussusception is an emergency. Go to the emergency room, or call 911.

The diagnosis is made by barium enema, and that is also the treatment.

If that does not solve the problem of bowel obstruction (pushing back the part of the intestine that is stuck), surgery is necessary.

Abdominal pain, painful and frequent urination. Abdominal pain, painful, burning urination, and frequent urination are signs of *urinary tract infection* (UTI).

The child can have fever as well.

The diagnosis is made by urine tests.

Treatment is medication.

(See urinary tract infection.)

Kidney stones (nephrolithiasis). This causes severe abdominal pain that radiates to the groin area. Bloody urine and vomiting are also frequent symptoms. Stone can be anywhere in the urinary tract.

The diagnosis is made by the history, the physical exam, a urine test, an x-ray (KUB), or a special x-ray called intravenous pyelography (IVP), an ultrasound or a CT scan—CT urography (see tests and procedures).

A urologist is involved in the child's care.

Treatment is fluid push, to help the stone to pass, lithotripsy to break the kidney stone by ultrasound shock waves to little pieces to avoid surgery. They can pass or be removed from the urinary tract. The last resort is surgery.

Often pain medication is needed.

Abdominal pain and constipation. Constipation often causes abdominal pain. It is important to know how often the child has bowel movements, and if they are normal or hard, and when was the last one.

If the pain is caused by constipation, the treatment is to stimulate the bowels. Change of diet, stool softener, laxative, or enema can help. However, if the child has vomiting as well, enema cannot be used.

With abdominal pain and constipation, the child needs to see the doctor (see constipation).

Abdominal pain, constipation, distended abdomen are the symptoms of *Hirschsprung disease* (see constipation).

If the abdominal pain is severe, the child had no stool for days, he or she vomits, and the abdomen is swollen, bowel obstruction can be the cause (see above).

That is a medical emergency. Go to the emergency room, or call 911.

Other diseases that can cause abdominal pain are strep throat, pneumonia, hepatitis, pelvic inflammatory disease (see sexually transmitted diseases), sickle cell disease (see anemia), gallstones (they are rare in children), ovarian cyst, ovarian torsion, twisted testicle, Henoch-Schönlein purpura, irritable bowel syndrome, and worms (see below).

Ovarian cyst, ovarian torsion. The ovaries are female reproductive organs located in the abdomen.

The ovaries grow cyst-like structures called follicles monthly. They produce hormones and release an egg when ovulation occurs, usually in the middle of the menstrual period. But if the follicle does not burst and does not release the egg, it continues to grow, becomes a cyst filled with fluid. This cyst often causes no symptoms and disappears in a few months.

But a large cyst can cause the ovary to twist, and the twisting of the ovary (ovarian torsion) cuts off the blood flow of the ovary that can cause damage of the organ.

Symptoms are severe abdominal pain, vomiting, and abdominal distention.

The diagnosis is made by ultrasound.

Urgent medical attention is needed. Go to the emergency room, or call 911.

Treatment is surgery.

Gynecologist is involved in the care of the girl if she has a cyst.

Twisted testicle (testicular torsion). This occurs when the testicle rotates, twisting the spermatic cord, and cuts off the blood supply of the testicle, causing permanent damage if not fixed in time.

Symptoms are suddenly developing pain in the scrotum and abdomen, swelling and extreme tenderness of the testicle, and vomiting.

The diagnosis is made by physical exam and sonogram.

If your child has the above symptoms, call 911.

Treatment is surgery as soon as possible.

Henoch-Schönlein purpura can cause severe abdominal pain.

Symptoms: The characteristic symptom is a rash. The rash consists of red spots. Some are small like pinpoints, but can be much larger. They do not disappear if you press them like a regular rash, because these are blood spots called purpura. The tiny pinpoint size spots are called petechiae. This rash is often seen on the legs and buttocks.

Abdominal pain that can be severe, painful swollen joints, and kidney involvement can be part of the clinical picture.

Henoch-Schönlein purpura usually goes away on its own, but kidney damage can occur.

If your child has a rash, abdominal pain, or joint pain, see the doctor.

Abdominal pain and vaginal bleeding

Ectopic pregnancy.
If a girl has vaginal bleeding, not related to her period, severe abdominal pain or severe pelvic pain, it can be ectopic pregnancy.

Ectopic pregnancy means that the pregnancy occurs outside the uterus, most often in one of the fallopian tubes (the two fallopian tubes carry eggs from the ovaries to the uterus).

Symptoms are severe abdominal or pelvic pain and vaginal bleeding. Extreme light-headedness, shoulder pain, and fainting can occur.

The diagnosis is made by a lab test and a sonogram. The lab test human chorionic gonadotropin (HCG) can confirm the pregnancy. The sonogram is the so-called transvaginal ultrasound. A device is placed into the vagina.

If the tube ruptures from the growing fertilized egg, heavy bleeding can happen in the abdomen. That creates an emergency situation because shock can develop (see change in consciousness, fast breathing, cold sweat—shock).

If a girl has severe abdominal pain and vaginal bleeding, that is an emergency. Go to the emergency room, or call 911.

A gynecologist will see the girl.

Treatment is surgery.

Chronic, recurrent abdominal pain. Chronic and recurrent abdominal pain is a complex problem, and often it is difficult to find the cause.

Important questions are mostly the same as with acute abdominal pain, but adding some more:

- Where is the pain located?
- How often has the child had the pain?
- How strong is the pain?
- Has anybody in the family had similar symptoms?
- Does the pain wake the child up at night?
- Is the pain related to eating?
- What does the stool look like?
- Is there any mucus or blood in the stool?
- Is the stool shiny as if it contains fat?
- Is it irregular and hard?
- Is there any vomiting or diarrhea?
- Is the urination okay?
- Are there any other complaints?

If the child has shiny stools with abdominal pain, the weight gain and growth slowed down, there is a suspicion of *celiac disease.* Celiac disease is sensitivity to gluten.

The diagnosis is made by history, physical exam, blood tests, and endoscopy with biopsy (see tests and procedures).

Treatment is a gluten-free diet (see diarrhea). The diagnosis should be made before a gluten-free diet is started.

Irregular hard stools can mean *chronic constipation,* and that often causes abdominal pain (see constipation).

Chronic abdominal pain, diarrhea, often with blood, are symptoms of *inflammatory bowel diseases (IBD): ulcerative colitis* and *Crohn's disease.*

Ulcerative colitis is the chronic inflammation of the large bowel (colon and rectum). *Crohn's disease* is chronic inflammation of the gastrointestinal tract.

Both diseases have symptoms of diarrhea that can be bloody, abdominal pain, and fatigue.

Both diseases can lead to anemia and weight loss. Complications can develop, like bleeding and dehydration. Symptoms of arthritis and inflammation in the eye, uveitis (see eye problems), can be present.

Laboratory tests, x-ray, and endoscopy (see tests, procedures, surgeries) help to make the diagnosis.

If the child has abdominal pain, bad diarrhea, or bloody stool, call the doctor.

The first line of treatment is steroids.

A gastroenterologist usually participates in the child's care.

A parasite, called *Entamoeba histolytica* also can cause bloody diarrhea, abdominal pain, fever, and weight loss. The name of the disease is *amebiasis*.

Contaminated food and water can transmit the disease.

The diagnosis is made from the stool.

Treatment is antiprotozoal medication, like metronidazole.

Meckel diverticulum can cause abdominal pain, with symptoms similar to acute appendicitis.

Meckel diverticulum is a bulge in the lower part of the small intestine. Meckel diverticulum is special because it has a mucus membrane like the stomach that secretes stomach acid. Meckel diverticulum is present at birth. It can be asymptomatic, or it can get inflamed, develop an ulcer, and bleed secondary to the acid. It also can cause perforation of the bowel, and bowel obstruction, including intussusception (see diarrhea).

The diagnosis is made by a radioactive scan.

Treatment is surgery.

Recurrent urinary tract infections can cause chronic abdominal pain. The symptoms of urinary tract infection are frequent, painful urination, dripping urine. Recurrent urinary tract infections are often associated with *vesicoureteral reflux* (VUR) (see urinary tract infection, UTI).

Stones in the urinary tract can also cause chronic abdominal pain (see above).

Chronic abdominal pain, vomiting, and tarry dark stools are symptoms of *peptic ulcer disease*. The pain usually occurs after eating. It can wake up the child at night. The ulcer can be located in the stomach or at the upper part of the small bowels (duodenum). A bacteria *Helicobacter pylory*, or *H. pylory*, can cause chronic inflammation that leads to the development of the ulcer. *H. pylori* can be detected from the stool, but the final diagnosis is made by endoscopy and biopsy.

The diagnosis of ulcer is made by x-ray, and/or endoscopy (a tube with a light is placed into the mouth and moved down into the stomach through the esophagus) (see tests, procedures, surgeries).

Complication of an ulcer can be bleeding and perforation. If bleeding, abdominal pain, and vomiting are present, urgent medical attention is needed. Go to the emergency room, or call 911.

If the child has abdominal pain, a gastroenterologist often participates in his care.

Treatment: Medications that decrease the acid production and medicine to treat the *H. pylori* infection. Severe complications from an ulcer as acute bleeding or perforation may require surgery.

Sometimes children with epilepsy can have stomachaches.

If the child has stomach pain at alternating places and no other symptoms are found, the pain can be secondary to stress.

Irritable bowel syndrome (IBS). Symptoms are abdominal pain, maybe increased number of stools, or change of the consistency of stools with the onset of pain. The pain can improve after bowel movement.

The physical exam is normal.

There is no laboratory test to make the diagnosis.

The diagnosis is made by the symptoms and by ruling out all other conditions causing abdominal pain.

Treatment is a diet rich in fibers, sometimes medications, and psychotherapy.

Worms can cause abdominal pain as well.

Hookworm, ascaris, and whipworm spread through contaminated soil.

Tapeworm and trichinella infect children by contaminated, incompletely cooked meat.

Diagnosis is made from stool samples.

Treatment is anthelmintic (treating infections caused by parasites) medication, like albendazole.

Stomachache (abdominal pain) always needs to be taken seriously, so your child should see the doctor.

But severe pain, vomiting, and swollen abdomen mean an emergency. Go to the emergency room, or call 911.

Substance abuse

Important questions:

- Has the behavior of the child or adolescent changed?
- Have his or her grades in school dropped?
- Has his or her absenteeism from school increased? How many days were missed?
- Does he or she have a new set of friends?
- Has the child stopped doing things that he or she liked to do before, like playing sports?

Stages of substance abuse:

- Stage 0—curiosity, risk-taking, desire to be accepted
- Stage 1—experimentation, weekend use, slight behavior change, lying
- Stage 2—regular use, mood swings, problems in school with declining grades and truancy, changing peer groups
- Stage 3—drug dependency, daily use, pathological lying, school failure, truancy, family fights, violence, driving under the influence
- Stage 4—using drugs to feel okay, all-day use, psychological changes can occur

Symptoms of paranoia, aggression, overdosing, blackout, and memory loss are common. The child has fatigue and malnutrition.

The consequence of overdose can be death.

When a child or adolescent is addicted to drugs, he or she will need more and more drugs to achieve the same effect as earlier with less drugs. At this stage, they are addicted, and they do anything to get the drug, including stealing and criminal activities.

Stage 0 and 1 is the best time to intervene.

Try to improve the child's self-esteem.

Establish strict but loving family guidelines.

Involve the child to participate in different activities, sports.

Try to get him or her away from friends who were a bad influence.

For the child who is on drugs already, the sooner the treatment begins, the better the chance is for success.

It is important to educate your child early on about the terrible dangers of drug use, and avoid people who use alcohol and drugs.

Substances that are often abused:

Alcohol. It causes stimulation first, then sedation, release of inhibitions. Other effects are red eyes, slurred speech, impaired balance and coordination—ataxia (see jerking and strange movements)—and impaired driving capability. Overdose causes poor judgment, impaired thinking, and emotional changes. Also decreased temperature, coma, and death can occur. Pregnant women's alcoholism can be deleterious for the baby—fetal alcohol syndrome (see agents that can harm the fetus). Alcohol abuse is responsible for many car accidents.

Cannabis, marijuana, weed. There is a misconception that the use of marijuana is not harmful.

Marijuana causes mild pleasant hallucinations, increased heart rate, and impaired abstract thinking and driving ability. Overdose causes acute anxiety. Regular use of marijuana can lead to mental and lung problems.

Cocaine. Cocaine can cause exhilaration, calmness, euphoria. But elevated temperature, irregular, fast heart rate and breathing, and high blood pressure can be present as well. Overdose can cause anxiety, elevated temperature, coma, and death.

Amphetamines. Amphetamines can cause stimulation, more energy, and decreased appetite. But overdose can cause irritability, paranoia, irregular heartbeats, hallucinations, and convulsions. Adderall is also an amphetamine.

Opiates (morphine, heroin, meperidine, methadone, fentanyl, hydrocodone, codeine, etc.). Their effects are drowsiness and euphoria. But slurred speech, unsteady walking, pinpoint pupils, and slower heartbeats and respirations are also the symptoms. Overdose can stop breathing. Many adolescents die from heroin overdose. Also, diseases like hepatitis B and human immunodeficiency virus (HIV) can be transmitted from person to person by shared needles.

The illegal drugs are made stronger and stronger; therefore, they are even more dangerous, like fentanyl. Recently, fentanyl can look like candy, and small amount (even one pill) can kill a child.

Hydrocarbons (glue, lighter fluid, gasoline fumes). They can cause excitement, slurred speech, impaired balance and coordination—ataxia (see jerking and strange movements)—double vision, and sleepiness. Death can occur. Chronic use can damage the lungs. Some users put a plastic bag over their head, and that can cause suffocation.

Hallucinogens like lysergic acid diethylamide (LSD). LSD causes vivid, colorful hallucinations. Dizziness, nausea, and fast heart rate and breathing are usual effects of LSD. Overdose causes panic reactions and terrifying hallucinations.

Phencyclidine (PCP)
Low dose produces euphoria. Higher doses can cause confusion, agitation, fast heart and respiratory rate, and distorted body perception. The adolescent can be combative or withdrawn. Overdose can cause seizures, very high blood pressure, brain hemorrhage, and death.

If you suspect that your child has a problem with drug abuse, call the doctor. Twenty-four-hour telephone hotline is also available to help. The telephone number of the Suicide and Crises Lifeline is 988.

If the child has a change of consciousness, agitation, hallucination, etc., urgent medical help is necessary. Go to the emergency room, or call 911.

If the child is addicted, treatment is necessary in a rehabilitation facility as soon as possible.

Tobacco smoking. Tobacco smoking is harmful, regardless of the vehicle that delivers it. Whether it is a cigarette, e-cigarette, or hookah smoking, all contain nicotine. E-cigarettes also have flavoring and solvents. They also can deliver other substances, including marijuana. Vaping or juuling is dangerous because it causes lung damage.

The "I quit ordinary smoking" (IQOS) heated tobacco is still smoking.

Smoking can cause chronic cough, bronchitis, chronic obstructive lung disease (COPD), and lung cancer in the long run. It can also cause problems with attention, learning, and mood change.

Children and adolescents care less about these consequences I just mentioned than how they look. Time seems to be limitless for them. Therefore, you can emphasize that tobacco smoke makes the teeth yellow, making him or her less attractive. Naturally, you also want to tell your child the more serious effects as well. Hopefully he or she will listen to that too.

Tobacco smoking of pregnant women can be very harmful for their baby. It can cause birth defects and sudden infant death syndrome (SIDS) (see agents that are harmful to the fetus).

Exposure to tobacco smoke as secondhand smoking is also harmful. Have your home and car smoke-free.

Swelling of the eyes, legs, and feet (edema)

Bug bites can cause swelling anywhere in the body, where there is soft tissue.

Allergic reactions can cause swelling, mostly at the eyes, lips, hands and feet.

Swelling of the eyelids can be caused by infection, as in case of periorbital cellulitis (see skin infections).

Swelling of the eyelids can be secondary to kidney disease.

Swelling of the eyes and legs can be manifestations of a certain kidney disease called *nephrotic syndrome* or nephrosis. In nephrotic syndrome, fluid can be accumulated in the abdomen too, causing swollen belly (abdominal distension from fluid, called ascites).

The urine contains much protein in this disease.

Treatment of nephrotic syndrome is steroid.

Low protein and low albumin level (albumin is a fraction of protein) in the blood is called *hypoproteinemia*. It can cause swelling anywhere in the body. The cause can be poor protein intake, or protein loss. Protein loss can be through the urine as in nephrotic syndrome, or through the gut from the so-called *protein losing enteropathy*.

Swelling of the legs and feet can also develop when the heart is unable to pump enough blood to the different parts of the body (*congestive heart failure*).

It can develop from a viral or bacterial infection. Rheumatic fever is caused by the bacteria group A *Streptococcus* if a strep throat or scarlet fever is not treated or not properly treated. Irregular heartbeats (arrhythmia) like in supraventricular tachycardia, high blood pressure, and congenital heart disease can cause congestive heart disease as well.

The symptoms of congestive heart disease are weakness, sweating, fast heart rate (tachycardia), fast breathing (tachypnea), and enlarged liver.

Diagnostic studies are x-ray, EKG (checking electrical impulses from the heart), echocardiogram (checking the structure of the heart by ultrasound).

Treatment is oxygen, fluid restriction, diuretics, and sometimes a drug called digitalis.

A heart doctor (cardiologist) is usually consulted.

In case of congenital heart disease, surgery might be necessary.

Heart problems can also develop secondary to respiratory distress or over-functioning thyroid gland (thyrotoxicosis). Obstructive sleep apnea also can cause heart problem. In those cases, the heart needs to work harder to keep up with the body's increased oxygen requirement (see heart problems).

Swelling of the legs and feet also can be secondary to injuries.

In all of these cases of swelling, medical attention is needed, except with minor trauma or minimal swelling around a bug bite. However, if there is also color change or trouble breathing, urgent medical attention is needed. Go to the emergency room, or call 911.

Swelling of the penis, testicle, and scrotum

Swelling of the tip of the penis is usually related to the *tightness of the foreskin—phimosis—*of uncircumcised boys. The inflammation is called *balanitis.* The symptoms are swelling, redness, pain, tenderness, and, often, discharge. The child may hold his urine because of pain with urination. If your son has these symptoms, he needs to see the doctor.

Treatment:

- Keep the area clean.
- Antibiotic ointment if needed.
- If the infection progresses and cellulitis develops, antibiotic therapy is necessary.
- Sometimes circumcision needs to be done.

For prevention, the boy needs to be taught good hygiene and how to clean the foreskin regularly.

Swelling of the foreskin and pain can develop if the foreskin gets stuck when it is pulled back (*paraphimosis*). If that happens, urgent medical attention is necessary because the skin can become necrotic. Go to the emergency room.

Treatment is the release of pressure by pulling the foreskin forward with the help of lubricants. But in certain cases, circumcision is necessary. Urologist is involved in the child's care.

The penis also can be swollen from bug bites. If there is swelling and redness, see the doctor.

Swelling of the testicle. Swelling of the testicle can be secondary to fluid accumulation (*hydrocele*). If it is found after birth, it usually resolves by one year of age. If it develops later, medical attention is needed.

Swelling, pain, and tenderness of the testicle raise the suspicion of *twisted testicle* (*testicular torsion*). Vomiting can develop too. This condition is an emergency. Go to the emergency room, or call 911.

A urologist will see the child.
Testicular torsion requires surgery. (See abdominal pain.)

Bug bites can cause the swelling of the scrotum.
Swelling of the scrotum can be caused by *hernia*.
Hernia develops if there is weakness of the abdominal wall, and the bowel moves to the scrotum through an opening, so hernia can develop at the groin area (inguinal hernia). Hernia can also develop at the thigh and at the navel. It is usually easy to place the bowel back through the abdominal wall.

Increased abdominal pressure from lifting, coughing, and sneezing can increase the size of the hernia. If the hernia gets painful, tender, and cannot be reduced, (incarcerated hernia), bowel obstruction may develop (see hernia). That is an emergency and needs surgery. Go to the emergency room, or call 911.

Swollen lymph nodes

Lymph nodes are part of the body's immune system, the fighting mechanism against infections. Normally, lymph nodes cannot be seen or palpated.

But if anywhere in the body there is an infection and inflammation, lymph nodes of that area become enlarged. The source can be insect bite, cut, sore, skin infection, or any infection of the deeper tissues. The cause of infection can be virus, bacteria, or fungus. The most common location of enlarged lymph nodes is the neck. After a sore throat, enlarged lymph nodes often can be found on the neck, mostly under the chin, on both sides.

Other places where enlarged lymph nodes are not uncommon are the armpit, the inguinal area, and the back of the head. The last one is a symptom of rubella (see infectious diseases of childhood).

Mononucleosis (*mono*) also causes enlarged lymph nodes on the neck (see mononucleosis).

Sometimes the source of an enlarged lymph node is not obvious. It can be only a solitary node, usually on the neck. In case of a bacterial infection, antibiotic treatment makes the node shrink or disappear. But also after a viral infection, the lymph node gets smaller, usually in about a couple of weeks. If the enlarged lymph node does not get smaller after a few weeks, and particularly if it gets bigger, further evaluation is necessary. That can include surgical removal of the node and analysis by a pathologist.

Parents sometimes accidentally find a small lymph node, and that makes them worry.

But in fact many children have small lymph nodes, mostly on their neck, without any problem.

They can be the remains of an old infection. They can get smaller or stay there forever.

Anyhow, enlarged nodes need to be checked by the doctor.

Cat scratch disease also causes enlarged lymph nodes (see cat scratch disease).

Teething, tooth and gum problems

Teething usually causes some discomfort but does not cause fever. Chewing on a cold teething ring can help to alleviate the pain. Do not use benzocaine for numbing your baby's or toddler's gum if teething or hurt, because if it is used under two years of age, methemoglobinemia can develop (see methemoglobinemia).

Babies usually start to get their first tooth around six months of age. Sometimes teething starts at four months. The twenty baby teeth or primary teeth are usually present by three years of age. The sequence of teething is generally the same. But there are exceptions, and that does not mean that the child has any problem. Most of the time, the two lower middle incisors erupt first. That is followed by the two upper middle teeth. Then two more upper and two more lower teeth come out in the middle. Next, the molars erupt around two years of age. Finally, the two upper and lower canines between the molars and the incisors come through.

To clean the baby's gum, initially you can use cloth and sterile water. When the teeth erupt, you can use a soft infant toothbrush and a tiny smear of toothpaste. At three to six years of age, you can use a pea-size toothpaste. Your child needs help with toothbrushing. Be sure he does not swallow the toothpaste.

Around ten years of age, he or she can use adult toothbrushes and toothpaste. Always use soft toothbrushes with a small head. The teeth need to be brushed twice a day.

Flossing the teeth is very important to prevent cavities. You can start flossing at two to three years of age and do it until your child is able to do it himself, around eight to ten years of age. Make flossing a positive experience so it becomes a habit like toothbrushing.

Tooth infection. Cavity (caries) is the most common tooth infection. It can be painful. If the cavity is not treated early on, the infection can spread to the root canal and surrounding tissues, and gum disease (*periodontitis*) can develop. Abscess (localized collection of pus) can be formed.

The prevention is good dental hygiene.

It is recommended to see the dentist every six months after six months to one year of age.

Fluoride is necessary to prevent cavities. Use fluoridated toothpaste. Communal water usually contains fluoride. If not, vitamins that include fluoride can be given. Fluoride can also be applied to the teeth (varnish). Discuss it with the doctor and dentist.

Too much fluoride though can cause mottling of the teeth.

Antibiotics like tetracycline or doxycycline can cause discoloration of the teeth. Therefore, they are not used before eight years of age (while the teeth are still developing) unless absolutely necessary.

To prevent the development of bad caries, be sure that the baby or toddler does not go to bed with a milk bottle. Also, your child should not eat or get any sweets after toothbrushing.

Embedded or impacted teeth are not erupted or only partially erupted.

Impacted teeth can get infected. There is swelling of the soft tissues in the area.

The child needs to see the dentist. Antibiotics are needed to treat the infection.

Tooth injury. If a tooth is injured, a dental appointment is necessary. If there is an avulsion of a tooth, put the tooth in saline solution, and get dental care as soon as possible, preferably within thirty minutes.

Gingivitis

Gingivitis is the inflammation of the gum.
Important questions are as follows:

- Is there any bleeding when your child brushes his teeth or flossing?
- Does his gum hurt?
- Is there any swelling of the gum?

Symptoms are bleeding, swelling, sores (ulcers) of the gum, pain, and bad breath.

Treatment and prevention are good dental hygiene with thorough toothbrushing and flossing.

If the symptoms are significant or do not improve, see the dentist.

Trench mouth (periodontal disease/periodontitis)

Trench mouth is a more severe form of gum disease (gingivitis) around the teeth.

It is caused by infection.

Symptoms are bleeding and swelling of the gum, pain, necrosis (ulcers), and bad breath.

A white, yellow, or green membrane can cover the ulcers.

Lymph nodes on the neck can be swollen and the child can have fever.

Treatment:

- Antibiotics
- Removal of the dead tissues
- Pain medications
- In severe cases, surgery could be necessary
- Periodontists treat gum diseases.

Thirst, drinking large amount of fluids, urinating much (diabetes mellitus, diabetes insipidus)

Thirst, drinking large amounts of fluids, and urinating too much indicates diabetes.

There are two types of diabetes: diabetes mellitus that is commonly called diabetes, and diabetes insipidus.

Diabetes mellitus means that the child has high blood sugar. It develops because the pancreas does not put out sufficient amounts of insulin to keep the blood sugar at normal level (insulin decreases the blood sugar).

In case of diabetes insipidus, either the pituitary gland does not produce enough antidiuretic hormone (ADH) or the kidneys do not respond to it. When the kidneys are making urine, the antidiuretic hormone pulls back water to the body, that way regulating the amount of urine.

Therefore, in diabetes insipidus, there is much fluid loss.

Diabetes mellitus. The hallmark is high blood sugar. There is type 1 and type 2 diabetes.

Type 1 diabetes is commonly called diabetes. Characteristic symptoms are thirst and drinking and urinating too much. The child often has weight loss. Often the first sign is bed-wetting and wetting the pants of a child who had been completely toilet-trained.

If the blood sugar is very high, the so-called *diabetic ketoacidosis* can develop. There is much fluid loss, and the child gets dehydrated (see dehydration). The symptoms are lethargy, dry, coated tongue, sunken eyes, and acetone smell. The urine contains sugar and ketones. Normal urine contains neither of them. The acids accumulate, and the child can lose consciousness. This is a serious condition, and without treatment, it can lead to coma.

Complications of diabetes mellitus are heart, kidney, eye diseases, and, often, nerve problems.

Treatment of diabetic ketoacidosis: intravenous (into the vein—IV) fluids and IV insulin.

Treatment of diabetes mellitus:

- Strict diet that regulates the intake of carbohydrates (sugar, sweet drinks, bread, pasta, pizza, tortilla, etc.).
- Exercise is very helpful to decrease blood sugar.
- Insulin under the skin (subcutaneous)
- The blood sugar needs to be monitored.

Type 2 diabetes

The blood sugar is high. Obesity is characteristic.

The color of the back of the neck is often black (*acanthosis nigricans*).

Symptoms are the same as in type 1 diabetes, and ketoacidosis can develop as well.

High blood pressure and high cholesterol are common in these children.

Treatment:

- Diet and exercise
- For symptomatic children, insulin and medications are available, but there is some insulin resistance, so insulin is less effective than in type 1 diabetes.

Diabetic children often have relatives with diabetes.

Diagnostic tests are blood sugar, urinalysis (the urine often has sugar), and hemoglobin A1c (HGB A1c) that shows the average blood sugar level for the past two to three months.

Regular checkups and daily monitoring of blood sugar is important.

Low blood sugar (*hypoglycemia*) secondary to insulin therapy can also be dangerous. Therefore, it is important that you and your child always have some sweet juice and/or candy at hand.

Children with diabetes usually need to see an endocrinologist. Diabetic ketoacidosis is an emergency, so go to the emergency room, or call 911.

Diabetes insipidus. Causes can be unknown, or diseases of the pituitary gland, like trauma, infection, tumor, can cause it, or problem with the kidneys, as mentioned above.

Symptoms are intense thirst, large amounts of urine output, fever, dehydration (see dehydration). Treatment is antidiuretic hormone. If a child has either diabetes mellitus or diabetes insipidus, an endocrinologist participates in the care of the child.

Typhus

Typhus is caused by bacteria called *Rickettsia*. Fleas and mites transmit the bacteria to humans. Typhus does not spread from person to person. It is rare in the US. Typhus can be severe.

Symptoms are fever, muscle pain, vomiting, rash, and change in mental status. Lymph nodes, liver, and spleen can be enlarged. If the child has a rash, it usually develops four to seven days after the disease develops.

Diagnosis is made by a blood test.

Treatment is an antibiotic doxycycline.

Undescended testicles (cryptorchidism)

The testicles can usually be palpated in the scrotum at birth. But rarely, a baby can have a condition called undescended testicle. That means that one or both testicles are not moved down from the abdomen to the scrotum through a tube in the groin (inguinal canal) and therefore not palpated in the scrotum at birth. This condition is more common in premature babies. Usually, one testicle is palpated at birth. The testicle still can move down to the scrotum in the first few months of life. However, if the testicle has not descended to the scrotum, the baby is usually referred to a urologist between six to twelve months of age.

There are also so-called *retractile testicles*, when the testicle is not in the scrotum, but it can be brought down from the inguinal canal.

Treatment of undescended testicles is surgery (orchiopexy). This procedure moves the undescended testicle into the scrotum and permanently fixes it there. That is important to prevent complications. The undescended testicle can affect fertility. It can also have malignant changes after some years.

Urinary tract infection (UTI)

The urine goes from the kidney to the ureter, then to the bladder and leaves the body through the urethra. This whole system is called the urinary tract. The infection of this system is called urinary tract infection (UTI). This means that the infection is somewhere in the urinary system but does not name a particular part of the system.

The most common bacteria causing UTI is *Escherichia coli* (*E. coli*). This germ can be found in the stool; therefore, girls are more susceptible to infection. Bacteria is carried over from the rectum to the urethra since they are in close proximity.

Important questions:

- Has the child been having painful urination? Is there a burning sensation with urination?
- Has the child been having frequent urination?
- Has the child been having problems urinating?
- Is the urine stream strong or weak? Is the urine dripping?
- After urination does the child feel that he needs to go again?
- The question for boys: Does he have a good urine curve?
- The question for girls: Does she have labial adhesion? (see below)
- Has the child been having abdominal, back, or side pain? If the answer is yes, does it radiate anywhere? Show where the pain is located.
- Is there any fever or vomiting?
- What does the urine look like? Is it dark or bloody?
- Does it have a foul odor?
- How often has the child been urinating? When was the last urine?
- For younger children: Is the child toilet-trained? If the answer is yes, has he or she had any accidents lately? If there are accidents, are they more frequent than usual?
- How often does the child have bowel movements? Are they normal, or are they hard? When was the last one?

- Has the child had urinary tract infection in the past?
- Is there anybody in the family who had urinary tract problems?

The symptoms of urinary tract infection are frequent and painful, often burning urination. Often the child has an urge to go to the bathroom, but when she gets to the toilet, she is unable to urinate, or the urine is only dripping. He or she may hold the urine because of the pain. Also, if the child is toilet-trained and starts to wet the bed, UTI is suspected. The urine can be dark and foul-smelling. If other symptoms like fever, vomiting, abdominal pain, or particularly flank pain develops, it can indicate an *infection of the kidneys—pyelone-phritis*. That requires immediate medical attention. Urgently see the doctor or go to the emergency room.

But to complain about these symptoms, the child needs to be old enough.

Infants and young children often cry, and their appetite decreases. They also often hold their lower abdomen. Fever, vomiting, and diarrhea can be present too.

However, a urinary tract infection can also develop insidiously without the above symptoms. Kidney stones predispose to UTI.

To make the diagnosis, the urine needs to be examined. That means that analysis of the urine, including microscopic exam, and urine culture (checking for bacteria) needs to be done. To do the urine culture, the urine is placed on a culture media, then to an incubator, and checked in twenty-four and forty-eight hours. If there is bacterial growth, it shows what bacteria is growing and how many colonies are there. The urine sample can be obtained by a catheter, and that is the most accurate method to collect the urine. The so-called bladder tap also provides sterile urine. After cleaning the skin, a needle is inserted to the bladder through the skin of the abdomen. Another less reliable but also less aggressive way to collect urine is called clean catch. In order to get a clean catch urine sample, the child needs to take a bath or a sitz bath (sitting in plain warm water). He or she needs to be cleaned with soap and water, then with antiseptic pads, usually three times. Children can urinate first a little to the toilet before getting the sample, and the rest of the urine goes to the urine cup. The urine of babies and toddlers is collected with a urine bag that is placed over the urethra. Again, this method is less reliable for urine culture.

If a baby or a child only has pain when urinating and no other symptoms are present, the cause can be from irritation or diaper rash.

Pinworms also can cause local irritation and skin damage because the child scratches the itchy skin.

Labial adhesions. Adhesions keep the inner lips (labia minora) of the girl's external genitalia closed. The attachment can be partial or full.

Labial adhesions usually occur in infants and young girls. Often there are no symptoms, but dribbling of the urine and frequent urinary tract infections can develop (see urinary tract infection [UTI]).

Labial adhesions often correct themselves at puberty, when more estrogen hormones are produced.

If treatment is necessary, usually a cream with estrogen is applied.

Good hygiene is important.

The treatment of urinary tract infection is antibiotic or other antimicrobial medicine.

When there are obvious and severe symptoms of a UTI present, your child might get antibiotics before the report of the urine culture is back. But if the bacteria is not sensitive to the antibiotic given, it will be changed. However, ideally the treatment starts after the urine culture identifies the germ causing the urinary tract infection and the sensitivity shows what antibiotic works best. The child also needs to drink plenty of fluids, including cranberry juice. Be sure to give the antibiotic regularly, and finish the whole course as prescribed by the doctor even if your child feels better after a few days.

If somebody has recurrent UTI, a disorder of the urinary tract can be suspected. The most common one is called *vesicoureteral reflux* (*VUR*). It means that not all the urine goes downward to the urethra and passes the body. Some urine will go upward, toward the kidneys. That way, the bacteria gets to the kidneys with the urine and causes an infection there. The infection of the kidney is called pyelonephritis, as mentioned above. VUR can cause kidney damage (scarring), from recurring infections. Therefore, the prevention of recurrent UTI is extremely important.

Preventative measures: girls should always wipe themselves from front to back, and they should not go back to the front with the same toilet paper.

It is helpful if you know your child's voiding habit, how often he or she goes to the restroom. Since infrequent urination makes the child susceptible to infections, have your child urinate at least every four hours.

It is also important to have normal bowel movements because constipation can play a role in the development of UTI.

Since children with reflux often have recurrent UTI, antibiotic prophylaxis may be necessary. That means that the child takes medicine daily until the reflux is resolved.

Reflux is graded according to what part of the urinary tract is reached by the urine. The lowest grade is I, when the urine reaches part of the ureter. The highest grade is V, when the urine gets to the kidney and causes urine retention and swelling there.

The diagnosis of reflux is done by x-ray, called voiding cysto-urethrogram (VCUG). When VCUG is done, a catheter is placed to the urethra, and contrast material is injected to the urinary tract. When the bladder is full and the child urinates, that is the time when the x-ray is done. If there is a reflux, the x-ray shows the urine going upward. Another method is the renal scan (radionuclide scan). It is usually done at yearly follow-ups since it exposes the child with less radiation than VCUG. However, it is less precise for grading reflux.

Kidney sonogram (renal sonogram) is also used to check the kidneys.

If a child has reflux, the urine needs to be checked every time when he or she has fever unless there is another obvious cause. If the child has recurrent infection, urine culture needs to be checked and antibiotic therapy given even if he or she was taking prophylactic antibiotics. A lower dose of antibiotic is given for prophylaxis than for therapy.

Children with reflux should see a urologist.

Most of the time, reflux will be resolved after a while (maybe years) without any intervention.

But in severe cases, surgery can be necessary.

Another treatment is Deflux therapy. Deflux is a gel-like bulking material that is injected to the wall of the bladder where the ureter is connected to the bladder using an instrument called cystoscope (see tests, procedures, surgeries).

Deflux forms a bulge there and works like a valve. The urine can flow into the bladder but not backward.

Posterior urethral valve. Posterior urethral valve is a membrane in the urethra. It is a rare birth defect that affects boys. It obstructs the urine flow through the urethra. The consequence is the dilation of the bladder, ureter, and kidney and possibly some damage.

Symptoms can be weak urine stream, difficulty with urination, and urinary tract infection.

Diagnosis is made with voiding cystourethrogram (VCUG).

Treatment is surgery.

All of these conditions are treated by urologists.

Vaginal discharge

It is important to check the color of the vaginal discharge. White discharge suggests yeast infection.

Yellow or green discharge is seen in bacterial infections.

Vaginal discharge is often caused by irritants like bubble bath, detergents, and fabric softeners. Yeast infection (monilia), foreign body, pinworms, poor hygiene also can cause discharge, itching, foul smell.

Sexually transmitted diseases can be the cause as well.

Prevention:

- No bubble bath. Use plain water and soap instead.
- Good hygiene.
- After using the toilet, wipe from front to back, and do not use the same paper again.

Viral infections

Adenovirus, coronavirus, Coxsackievirus, enterovirus, Epstein-Barr virus, herpesvirus, arbovirus, influenza virus, parainfluenza virus, rhinovirus, metapneumovirus, norovirus, rotavirus, respiratory syncytial virus (RSV), HIV virus

Viruses also cause chickenpox, measles, mumps, rubella, poliomyelitis or polio, roseola, fifth disease (see infectious diseases of childhood).
Mosquito-transmitted diseases are also caused by viruses.

Arboviruses. These cause chikungunya, dengue, West Nile, Zika virus diseases (see mosquito transmitted diseases).

Adenovirus. This can cause symptoms of a cold, but more severe diseases can develop as well. It can cause tonsillitis (see sore throat), ear infection, pink eye, bronchiolitis, or even pneumonia and meningitis.

Coronavirus. This can cause symptoms of runny nose, cough, and pink eye. Coronavirus also can cause severe pneumonia, as in severe acute respiratory syndrome (SARS), or in the Middle East respiratory syndrome (MERS), or in the recent novel coronavirus infections (*COVID-19* pandemic).
This virus is very contagious, and new variants (mutations) can appear like Omicron.
Symptoms may develop two to fourteen days after exposure to the virus.
Symptoms: fever, chills, runny nose, cough, sore throat, loss of smell, shortness of breath, fatigue, headache, body aches, muscle pain, vomiting, and diarrhea. Tests are available to diagnose COVID-19 infections.
The virus most often attacks the lungs but can affect any part of the body.

It affects children as well and can cause severe disease—*multisystem inflammatory syndrome (MIS-C)*.

Symptoms of MIS-C: fever for a few days, rash, red eyes, red chapped lips, enlarged lymph nodes, swelling of hands, feet, joint pain, extreme weakness, severe headache, change of consciousness, difficulty breathing, vomiting, and diarrhea. If your child has any of these symptoms, call the doctor.

If your child has trouble breathing, color change (lips turning bluish), change of consciousness, or any other severe symptoms, call 911. Let the operator know that the child probably has COVID-19.

Precautions for COVID-19:

- Wear mask in closed public places.
- Keep social distancing (six feet).
- Prefer being outside if weather permits.
- Have your child sneeze and cough into a disposable tissue covering the nose and mouth, or a flexed elbow.
- Good hygiene is always important not only in the time of a pandemic. Teach this to your child early on.
- Most of all have your child immunized with a COVID-19 vaccine. COVID-19 is added to the immunization schedule in 2023. It is available for children after 6 months of age.
- Children can have long COVID too.
- Follow the guidelines issued by the Centers for Disease Control and Prevention (CDC) and your local health department.
- Children with COVID need to be quarantined.
- Monoclonal antibodies and new antiviral drugs are available to treat COVID-19 infections.

Enteroviruses. These *are:* coxsackieviruses, echoviruses, and poliovirus.

Coxsackie virus can cause sores in the mouth. But sores also can appear on the hands, feet, and often on the buttocks. This illness is called *hand, foot and mouth disease*. The child usually has a fever. Fluid intake is limited because of the pain, so the child can get dehydrated. Therefore, it is important to give him plenty of fluids. Do not give juices or anything irritating. Tylenol can be given for pain.

Heart disease caused by coxsackie virus B can be severe.

Echoviruses, like other enteroviruses, can cause illnesses with fever, runny nose, sore throat, vomiting and diarrhea, but also can cause diseases such as bronchiolitis, pneumonia, heart disease (myocarditis) and neurologic disease (meningitis).

Polio virus is also an enterovirus. It is an infection of the spinal cord and brain.

The infected child can have no or mild symptoms or a severe disease. The name of the disease is poliomyelitis (polio).

Symptoms: Fever and headache. If vomiting and stiff neck is present too, meningitis is suspected (see vomiting).

This virus can cause so called paralytic polio with weakness then paralysis of different muscles.

It can cause difficulty breathing secondary to the paralysis of muscles necessary for breathing. But also the breathing center of the brain (brain stem) can be affected.

No therapy exists, but prevention is available in the form of vaccination (IPV, oral polio). IPV is part of the immunization schedule.

Thanks to the vaccines, the disease is eradicated in most countries including the USA. The importance of immunization against polio is underlined by the fact that a person who has not been immunized became sick with polio in the US in 2022.

Epstein-Barr virus. This causes mononucleosis or mono (see mononucleosis).

Hepatitis viruses. These cause liver disease, hepatitis (see hepatitis).

Herpes infections. The herpes simplex virus causes blisters and sores at the site of infection.

There are two types of herpes simplex virus (HSV). Herpes simplex virus 1 (HSV1) causes cold sores and fever blisters on and around the lips and in the mouth.

Herpes simplex 2 (HSV2) causes genital herpes.

When the child gets blisters in the mouth, it is called *herpetic gingivostomatitis.*

It is contagious, transmitted by the saliva. The blisters are painful, and the child might refuse to drink because of the pain. That can lead to dehydration. Fever is also present.

The fever blisters can recur. Fever, cold, and sunburn are the most common triggers. It usually resolves in a week.

Treatment: Antiviral ointment (Acyclovir) can shorten the course. If the blisters are located in the mouth, pain medications Acetaminophen (Tylenol) or Ibuprofen (Motrin, Advil) can be given. If the blisters are not on the throat, sometimes anesthetic drops are used locally for the pain. The child should not swallow it. Be sure that your child drinks enough fluids. Call the doctor. Herpesvirus also can affect the eyes, causing so called keratitis (see eye problems).

An ophthalmologist treats the child with keratitis.

Herpes simplex virus may affect the thumb in thumb-suckers.

Herpes also can affect different organs. *Inflammation of the brain (encephalitis)* is the most severe.

Herpes virus—genital herpes. Genital herpes is a sexually transmitted disease (STD).

The cause is mostly herpes simplex virus type 2, but sometimes type 1.

Blisters and sores develop at the genital area. They are painful, spontaneously resolve, but can recur.

Transmission of the herpes virus from the mother to the newborn is frequent, even when the mother has no symptoms but is infected. Herpes is a very dangerous disease in newborns. The baby looks okay after birth but develops symptoms in a few days. Fever or very low temperature, feeding problems, irritability or lethargy, breathing problems or convulsions can develop. The disease can leave devastating consequences, mostly because the brain is involved (encephalitis). (See agents that harm the fetus.)

Treatment for the mother is oral. For the baby is IV antiviral medicine, like Acyclovir.

Many viruses can cause common cold or upper respiratory infection (URI).

Influenza. This can cause epidemics.

Parainfluenza. This causes similar symptoms as influenza virus does.

Metapneumovirus. This can cause upper respiratory infection, bronchiolitis, croup, and pneumonia.

Norovirus. This often causes diarrhea with fever and vomiting. Outbreaks have occurred.

Transmission happens from contaminated food and drink, but the disease also spreads from person to person (see diarrhea).

Rotavirus. This causes diarrhea that can be severe, with dehydration. Since the introduction of the rotavirus vaccine, the number of cases has decreased (see diarrhea).

Respiratory syncytial virus (RSV). RSV virus causes wheezy bronchitis, bronchiolitis. It can cause breathing problems (see cough, respiratory problems, respiratory distress).

In general, there is no need to know what kind of virus causes the given illness.

However, sometimes the virus needs to be identified. In that case, the laboratory tests are done from the nose, throat, and rectum.

No specific therapy exists to treat most of these viral infections. Usually medications are given to decrease the fever. After six years of age, sometimes cold medications are given to decrease the symptoms. Plenty of fluids and rest are recommended.

If the symptoms are significant, or fever is present for over a day, see the doctor. However, if a baby has fever, he or she needs to be seen by the doctor on the same day when the fever developed. If the child has shortness of breath, vomiting, or lethargy, go to the emergency room, or call 911. Babies with fever under three months of age, children with fever above 104 degrees Fahrenheit, and if the child has no urine for nine to ten hours should go to the emergency room. If your child has fever, give him fever reducer before you go to the emergency room.

The child can go back to school if no fever is detected for twenty-four hours.

Preventative measures are good handwashing and avoiding close contact with sick persons. Premature babies can receive antibodies for prevention to fight RSV infection (Synagis) a monoclonal antibody nirsevimab is a new tool for prevention. There is an RSV vaccine available for pregnant women to protect the baby.

Yearly influenza shots are recommended for everybody above six months of age.

HIV infection, acquired immunodeficiency syndrome (AIDS). HIV-infected mothers can transmit the infection to their newborns. The child with HIV has a weakened immune system and has a decreased capability of fighting infections. He or she can have frequent severe or rare infections and cancer. They can have enlarged lymph nodes, an enlarged liver and spleen, and weight loss.

Treatment is antiretroviral therapy. (See agents that can harm the fetus.)

Common cold or "flu"—upper respiratory infection (URI) and influenza. "Common cold" is a collective name for viral infections that can be caused by different viruses. Upper respiratory infection is another name for it.

But the common cold is also often called flu. That is confusing because influenza is also called flu. There is another confusion, because there is a bacteria called *Haemophilus influenzae* or *H. flu*. Common cold and the influenza are infections caused by viruses. Since *H. flu* is a bacteria, only the name is similar.

Influenza can be type A, B, and C. Type A and B are significant, causing severe diseases and often epidemics. Type C causes only sporadic and mild disease.

Influenza appears yearly, mostly in the fall, winter, and spring.

In certain years, the influenza virus causes serious disease all around the world (pandemic).

The incubation period for both influenza and the common cold is a few days.

The symptoms are similar for both influenza and common cold—fever, runny nose, sneezing, coughing, sore throat. Pink eyes and headaches are common.

But if a child has influenza, he or she is very tired and has body aches as well. Influenza can also cause vomiting and diarrhea. Since both influenza and the common cold are viral illnesses, antibiotics do not help, unless a bacterial superinfection develops.

Complications can develop with both influenza and the common cold. They mostly cause ear infection, sinus infection, croup, laryngitis, bronchitis, bronchiolitis, and pneumonia.

Medications like fever reducers (acetaminophen, ibuprofen), cold medicines, and nasal sprays can alleviate some symptoms. Do not use Afrin Nasal spray longer than three days. Do not give cold medications to your child if he or she is younger than six year. Plenty of fluids and rest are recommended.

The child needs to stay at home. There are antiviral medications to treat influenza (oseltamivir, zanamivir). These medications can also be used for prophylaxis.

For the prevention of both influenza and the common cold, good handwashing is important. During influenza season, try to avoid crowds.

Sick persons with sneezing and cough should cover their nose and mouth. Try to avoid close contact with them until they are better. For the prevention of influenza, people who are exposed can also get antiviral medications.

Influenza vaccines are the mainstay of prevention. The influenza virus has the capability to change, so the vaccine given last year most likely does not work this year. Therefore, the vaccine is also changing every year.

Do not give aspirin if your child has influenza, chickenpox, or any other viral disease. It can lead to the development of a serious condition called Reye's syndrome. Symptoms of the disease include vomiting, change of mental status, confusion, and delirium. There is liver damage and effects on the brain.

Rhinoviruses frequently cause common cold (URI).

Vitamins

Vitamins are necessary to keep the body functioning normally.

There are fat-soluble vitamins, Vitamin A, D, E, K, and water-soluble vitamins, Vitamin C and vitamin B complexes.

Excess intake of fat-soluble vitamins can cause harm (see chapter on poisonings).

Vitamin A. Food sources: liver, carrots, fish liver oil, milk, eggs, broccoli, cantaloupe, beans, sweet potatoes, lettuce.

Deficiency symptoms: night blindness, dryness of the eyes (xerophthalmia), decreased resistance to fight infections.

Vitamin B complex

Vitamin B 1 (thiamine). Food sources: Yeast, whole grain, brown rice, cereal.

Vitamin B1 deficiency causes a disease called *beriberi.*

Symptoms: weakness, muscle wasting, problem walking, burning sensation from nerve dysfunction (neuropathy). It also can cause cardiac problems.

Vitamin B2 (riboflavin)

Food sources: meat, eggs, dairy, green vegetables, fortified cereals.

Deficiency symptoms: sores on the sides of the lips (cheilosis), inflammation of the tongue (glossitis) and the mouth (stomatitis), and poor growth.

Vitamin B3 (niacin)

Food sources: meat, eggs, beans, fortified cereals.

Vitamin B3 deficiency causes a disease called pellagra.

Symptoms: skin irritation (dermatitis), diarrhea, mental dullness, memory impairment (dementia) The sun exposed skin gets red, blisters develop, then the skin gets rough, hard, and scaly.

Vitamin B6. Food sources: Fish, milk, eggs, yeast, banana, fortified cereals.

Deficiency symptoms are similar to Vitamin B2 deficiency. Vitamin B6 deficiency rarely can cause seizures in infants.

Vitamin B12 (cobalamin). Food sources: Liver, meat, fish, eggs, milk, cheese, yeast, fresh green vegetables.

Vitamin B12 deficiency causes pernicious anemia.

Symptoms: anemia, the red blood cells are large (macrocytic megaloblastic anemia).

It also can cause neurological problems like muscle weakness, mental dullness, memory loss. Vision problems can be present as well.

Vitamin C (ascorbic acid). Food sources: fresh fruits and vegetables.

Vitamin C deficiency causes a disease called *scurvy.*

Symptoms: bleeding of the gums, but bleeding can develop anywhere in the body.

Vitamin D. Food sources: fish, liver, eggs, fortified milk. The skin exposed to sunlight produces vitamin D.

Vitamin D deficiency causes a disease called *rickets.*

Symptoms: poor appetite, weakness, and softness of the skull (craniotabes) in babies. Children also have bow leg and tooth defects. It also can cause low calcium levels in the blood (hypocalcemia). Symptoms of very low calcium levels are muscle spasms. It can be painful. Spasm in the larynx can cause breathing difficulty (laryngospasm). Seizure can occur too.

Diagnosis is made by lab tests and x-ray.

Vitamin E. Food sources: cereal, seed oils, peanuts, soybean, milk.

Vitamin E deficiency can cause a type of anemia, when some red blood cells get destroyed, called hemolytic anemia (see anemia).

Vitamin K. Food source: liver, milk, green leafy vegetables.

Deficiency: It can cause bleeding; therefore, Vitamin K is given to newborns for prevention. It also can cause neurologic disorders.

Folic acid. Food sources: liver, cereal, green vegetables, oranges.

Deficiency: It can cause anemia that is similar to the one that is caused by Vitamin 12 deficiency. There are some immature and dysfunctional red blood cells, called megaloblasts. It also can cause growth failure, delayed maturation of the nervous system, diarrhea, inflammation of the tongue, and sores in the mouth.

Folate deficiency in pregnant women increases the risk of birth defects. Therefore, pregnant women need to take folate, but it should not be more than the dose recommended by the obstetrician.

The treatment of all the vitamin deficiencies is vitamin supplement as recommended by the doctor.

The prevention of vitamin deficiencies is a diet rich in vitamins (see the specific foods above with each vitamin).

Too much vitamin A and D can be harmful (hypervitaminosis. See poisoning).

Vomiting

As mentioned earlier, there is a common belief that a child is only sick if he or she has fever. But another symptom, at least as important, is vomiting.

Babies often spit up food, but only a small amount, one or two teaspoons or a tablespoon, and it does not come out with force.

If the baby spits up but is happy and otherwise doing well and gaining weight, that is normal.

If the amount of food coming out is larger than a spit-up, it is vomiting. But if the vomiting is large and comes up with force, that is projectile vomiting.

It is important to distinguish what kind of vomiting a child has.

- Is it spitting up?
- Is it vomiting?
- Is it projectile vomiting?
  Important questions:
  - How many times did the child vomit?
  - Has he had projectile type vomiting?
  - How does the vomiting look like?
  - What is the color?
  - Is there any blood in it?
  - Is it yellow or foul smelling?
  - Does the child have diarrhea, fever, stomachache, or swollen abdomen?

Vomiting is important because it can be a symptom of a severe disease, and it also can lead to dehydration, regardless of the cause.

During the first year of life, any disease can cause vomiting. A good example is ear infection.

The vomiting is particularly severe if the child cannot keep even small amounts of water down.

If vomiting occurs more than twice in a row, it is considered to be significant, and the doctor needs to be called.

When vomiting is the only symptom. If a baby spits up frequently, sometimes vomits and is losing weight, reflux (gastroesophageal reflux) is a good possibility. The milk goes from the stomach back to the esophagus and the mouth. If it happens regularly and significantly, it is called *gastroesophageal reflux disease* (*GERD*). If the food comes back and gets to the airways (aspiration), coughing, choking, and infection of the lung, pneumonia, can be the consequence. If this event happens regularly, chronic cough can develop, as well as bronchitis, bronchiolitis, and pneumonia.

Older children with reflux will complain of heartburn. Other symptoms are chest pain, burping, getting food into the mouth, stomachache, vomiting, gagging, coughing, and slow weight gain.

The diagnosis is made by the history and physical exam.

If the reflux causes complications, x-ray, barium swallow, endoscopy, and esophageal manometry are the diagnostic options (see tests, procedures, surgeries).

Treatment for babies:

- Avoid feeding too much at one time.
- Increase burping time.
- Feed with thickened formula.

For babies and children, medications like Prevacid are available. These medications suppress the acid secretion of the stomach (ranitidine Zantac has been removed from the market).

Treatment for children:

- Avoid large meals before exercise and bedtime.
- The child needs to stay upright for three hours after eating.
- Limit the amount of food that could make reflux worse, like sodas with caffeine, chocolate, fried foods, oranges and tomatoes.
- If these measures do not help, antacids like Mylanta or other medications like Pepsid or Prevacid can be tried.

Uncomplicated reflux does not need treatment with medications. If the reflux is mild, the baby usually grows out of it. Medications are needed in the following:

- If there is poor weight gain (failure to thrive).
- If other measures did not work.
- If endoscopy shows the inflammation of the esophagus.
- If a child has reflux and asthma.

Children with very severe GERD might need surgery.

Between two weeks and two months of age, a baby with frequent or continuous projectile vomiting is suspected to have so-called *pyloric stenosis*. In that condition, the stomach muscle is thickened and blocks the passage of food.

It often leads to dehydration.

The diagnosis is made by clinical signs and ultrasound or x-ray. CT scan, ultrasound, and barium enema can help to make the diagnosis.

The treatment is surgery.

If an older child vomits once or twice, and after that he or she feels fine, has no other complaints or symptoms, the cause can be overeating or having something that did not agree with the child's stomach. The child feels better after vomiting. If there is no more vomiting, the problem is solved. Keep a clear liquid and BRAT diet (see diarrhea) for a day or so.

Some other causes of vomiting are gastroenteritis (see diarrhea), food allergy (see allergies: allergic reaction, food poisoning (see diarrhea), migraine (see headache), motion sickness (see motion sickness).

Vomiting and cough. Strong cough can cause vomiting. Also coughing with phlegm can cause nausea and then vomiting. Babies and young children cannot spit up mucus. They swallow it, and vomiting is the way to get rid of the phlegm. Postnasal drip from a sinus infection also can cause nausea and vomiting (see sinus infections).

Whooping cough can cause coughing spells and vomiting. It is less common than it used to be thanks to immunizations, but it is still around. Therefore, it is important for mothers and caretakers to have their current Tdap shot for the protection of the baby they care for (see infectious diseases of childhood).

Coughing spells and vomiting occur often with bronchiolitis, reactive airway disease, and asthma. Wheezing is often part of the picture (see cough, respiratory problems, respiratory distress).

Vomiting and swollen belly (abdominal distention). Severe vomiting and swollen belly can be signs of a severe condition, *bowel obstruction.* This is the blockage of the small or large intestine. Bowel obstruction can occur soon after birth or later in life (see stomachache).

The symptoms are vomiting, swollen belly, and lack of bowel movements. Children also experience abdominal pain and tenderness.

Diagnosis is made by the symptoms, physical exam, and x-ray.

Treatment is surgery most of the time. The use of a nasogastric tube (a tube is placed to the stomach through the nose) and intravenous fluids (fluids given through the vein) are also necessary.

Severe vomiting and swollen belly needs urgent medical attention. Go to the emergency room, or call 911.

Bowel perforation causes the same symptoms as bowel obstruction. The diagnostic tools are the same. Treatment is surgery (see stomachache).

Acute pancreatitis also can cause an acute abdomen (see stomachache).

Symptoms are abdominal pain, vomiting, fever. The belly is often swollen (distended) and tender.

The diagnosis is made by the clinical picture and laboratory tests, showing elevation of the enzymes of the pancreas, amylase and lipase.

Treatment consists of IV fluids and nasogastric tube.

Hirschsprung disease (see constipation).

Vomiting and hernia. When a child has a hernia, there is a lump present, most often at the groin area, rarely at the thigh. If the lump is tender and cannot be pushed back easily to the inguinal canal, and the child is screaming and vomiting, bowel obstruction can be present, caused by a so-called *incarcerated hernia.*

This is an emergency. Go to the emergency room, or call 911.

Vomiting and diarrhea. These two symptoms are often seen together. If a child has both vomiting and diarrhea, that means he or she has *gastroenteritis,* the inflammation of the stomach and bowels.

The cause most often is viral or bacterial infection.

The important thing is to be sure that the child does not have significant fluid loss (dehydration). Babies become dehydrated faster than older children. The more frequent the vomiting and diarrhea are, and the larger the amount is, the risk of dehydration is higher because there is more fluid loss. You want to be able to tell the doctor how much vomiting or diarrhea your child has and how it looks. You also need to notice whether the vomiting was projectile or not and what the color was. It is very important to notice if the vomit was yellow or foul-smelling (smelling like stool) because that can indicate a bowel obstruction.

Vomiting, bloody diarrhea, and stomach cramps. While these symptoms can occur if a child has severe gastroenteritis, they are also present in case of a serious condition called *intussusception.* In this case, part of a bowel slides into another part of the bowel, causing obstruction.

It usually occurs in infancy and early childhood.

Symptoms are severe periodic abdominal cramps, causing the child to scream, vomiting, then bloody stool with mucus, and distended, tender abdomen. Fever can develop. Bowel sounds are absent.

The diagnosis is made by x-ray, barium enema (an enema is given with a contrast material called barium).

Treatment:

- Nasogastric tube
- IV fluids
- Barium enema. (See abdominal pain.)
- Surgery (if the barium enema does not solve the problem)

This is an emergency. Go to the emergency room, or call 911.

Vomiting, fever, abdominal pain.
The above symptoms can indicate *appendicitis* (see stomachache).

Vomiting and fever. Vomiting and fever are symptoms of many diseases, most often infections.

You need to take your child to the doctor to find out the cause.

Vomiting, fever and lethargy. High fever, projectile vomiting, and lethargy raise the suspicion of a serious disease, meningitis. *Meningitis* is an infection of the membranes around the brain.

It is most often caused by viruses or bacteria. Bacterial meningitis is more severe.

Symptoms are vomiting, lethargy, fever. The baby's soft spot is bulging.

The diagnosis is likely if the child has a stiff neck, but it is only confirmed by spinal tap, also called lumbar puncture. A needle is inserted to the spinal canal, draining out a small amount of spinal fluid to be sent to the laboratory for analysis and culture.

The treatment of bacterial meningitis (meningitis caused by a germ) is a combination of intravenous antibiotics.

Encephalitis is an inflammation in the brain and is usually caused by viruses.

The child can have meningitis at the same time (meningoencephalitis).

Symptoms are the same as in meningitis, and the diagnosis is made the same way as well.

Treatment is dependent on the symptoms.

If vomiting, fever, and lethargy are present, urgent medical attention is necessary. Go to the emergency room, or call 911.

Vomiting and head trauma. In case of head trauma, the important questions are the following:

- Has the child had loss of consciousness? Does he or she remember what happened?
- Has the child had projectile vomiting (vomiting with force)?
- Was he or she able to walk normally, or was the walk wobbly?
- Was there any dizziness or headache?
- Is there any vision problem?

In case of head trauma and vomiting, urgent medical attention is needed.

Go to the emergency room, or call 911. However, in case of severe head trauma, just call 911. Turn the whole body to the side to avoid aspiration (accidentally breathing in foreign material) from vomitus. Do not move the head because neck injury is very possible.

Warts

Warts are skin-colored growths. They are rough to the touch and occur most often on the fingers and hand but can grow any-where on the skin.

The cause is a virus, human papillomavirus (HPV) and is trans-mitted by touch.

Take your child to the doctor if the growth is painful, if the appearance, the border of the wart, or the color changed, and if you are not sure whether it is a wart.

It can be treated locally with medicine, such as salicylic acid, or freezing but can also be removed by a doctor, often a skin doc-tor (dermatologist). It can also disappear spontaneously after a long time.

Genital warts (condyloma acuminata) is spread by sexual con-tact (see sexually transmitted diseases).

Weakness, sweating, hunger, tremor (hypoglycemia)

The above symptoms suggest the presence of *low blood sugar* (*hypoglycemia*).

Mood and personality change are not uncommon during an episode of low blood sugar, and loss of consciousness can occur. Extremely low blood sugar can be life-threatening.

Causes: Low blood sugar is not uncommon in newborns. Premature babies and newborns whose weight is less than 10 percentile on the growth chart are more prone to low blood sugar. Mothers who have diabetes usually have large babies, and those are also at higher risk for low blood sugar.

Children with diabetes can have low blood sugar because they receive too much insulin, and that can lower their blood sugar too much.

Some *metabolic and endocrine problems* can also cause low blood sugar.

Treatment: If the child is conscious, he or she needs to drink sugar containing drinks, like sodas or juices. If your child has diabetes, always have some sweets with you.

If the consciousness is altered, or the child is unconscious, call 911. Intravenous fluid that contains sugar needs to be given.

It is important to recognize the symptoms early on, so the development of serious symptoms can be prevented.

3

Tests, Procedures, Surgeries, and Health-Care Professionals

Tests

Blood tests. Complete blood count (CBC) measures the number of white blood cells, red blood cells, and platelets.

High or very low white blood cell count suggests infection.

Low red blood cell count means anemia.

Platelet count shows if the count is high enough for normal blood clotting. Low count is a risk for bleeding.

Prothrombin time (PT) measures how quickly the blood clotting occurs in a blood sample.

Partial thromboplastin time (PTT) evaluates coagulation factors.

Fibrinogen is a protein necessary for blood clotting. This test shows the fibrinogen level in the blood.

Hemoglobin analysis is done by a method called electrophoresis. This test can analyze the hemoglobin in the red blood cells. It is used to identify abnormal hemoglobin, like in sickle cell anemia.

Sedimentation rate (sed rate or ESR) shows how quickly the red cells sediment. It checks for inflammation in the body. If the child has an infection, the ESR is usually elevated.

C-reactive protein (CRP) is also checking for inflammation and infection. In case of infection, it is usually elevated.

Procalcitonin is a marker to check for infection and inflammation.

Antistreptolysin O (ASO) test: If the titer is elevated, it suggests a recent infection with group A *Streptococcus*.

Rheumatoid factor helps to diagnose juvenile idiopathic arthritis (JIA).

Antinuclear antibody test (ANA) helps in the diagnosis of autoimmune diseases like lupus erythematosus.

Tests for mononucleosis: monospot is a screening test.

Epstein-Barr (EBV) antibodies show infection with the EB virus that causes mononucleosis.

Comprehensive metabolic panel (CMP): It measures the electrolytes, carbon dioxide, calcium, blood sugar, blood urea nitrogen (BUN), serum creatinine, and liver enzymes. It also shows the bilirubin level and serum protein. The electrolytes and calcium are vital for the normal functioning of the body. BUN reflects on hydration and kidney function. Creatinine reflects on the kidney function as well. Bilirubin, alanine transaminase (ALT), aspartate aminotransferase (AST), and alkaline phosphatase reflect on the function of the liver. CMP measures also the total serum protein and its fractions, albumin and globulin. The serum protein (mostly albumin) keeps the fluid in the blood vessels. So if it is low (hypoproteinemia), swelling develops in different parts of the body (see swelling of the eyes, legs, feet). Globulin is needed for the immune system. The albumin to globulin ratio is measured, and if it is elevated, it suggests infection. The carbon dioxide or bicarbonate shows the body's acid base balance. In severe dehydration, there is acidosis, and the bicarbonate is low.

Blood sugar (BS) measures the glucose level in the blood. Elevated blood sugar suggests diabetes mellitus (see thirst, drinking large amounts of fluids, urinating much) low blood sugar can cause problems as well (see sweating, hunger, tremor (hypoglycemia).

The hemoglobin A1c test reflects a person's average blood sugar level in the past two to three months.

Liver enzymes show if the liver functions are normal (see above).

Lipid profile: it shows the level of triglycerides and cholesterol in the blood, including the level of the high-density lipoprotein

(HDL), the "good" cholesterol, and low-density (LDL), the "bad" cholesterol (see obesity).

Sweat chloride test measures the chloride concentration of the child's sweat. High chloride content is diagnostic to cystic fibrosis (see cough, respiratory problems, respiratory distress).

Vitamin D test shows the level of vitamin D in the blood. Low level means vitamin D deficiency. In that case, a vitamin supplement is needed (see vitamins).

Hormone levels can be checked, like growth hormone, thyroid hormones, etc.

Urine tests. Urinalysis is the analysis of the urine by a urine test strip. It checks the so-called specific gravity concentration of urine, looks for white blood cells (leukocytes), red blood cells (RBC), screens for nitrate, urobilinogen, protein, pH, blood, ketones, bilirubin, and glucose.

Specific gravity and ketones reflect on the child's hydration.

Leukocytes and nitrates check for kidney infection. Blood and protein in the urine can indicate other kidney problems.

Urobilinogen and bilirubin screen for liver problems.

Checking the sugar in the urine screens for diabetes.

The pH and ketones reflect on the acid content of the body.

Cultures. There are bacterial, viral, and fungus cultures. They check for the specific bacteria, virus, or fungus that is causing a given infection. They are done from body fluids, excretions, and discharges.

The most common cultures are urine, stool, and blood.

Laboratory tests help the doctor to make the diagnosis. But they are never substitutes for the history, physical exam, and medical decision-making.

QuantiFERON-TB Gold test (interferon-gamma release assay or IGRAs). This helps to diagnose tuberculosis (TB) (see cough; respiratory problems, respiratory distress).

Tuberculin test or Mantoux test is another test for the diagnosis of tuberculosis. This is a tiny shot. A small amount of fluid called tuberculin is pushed into the skin of the forearm with a syringe and needle, making a small bump. The child's arm needs to be looked at in forty-eight to seventy-two hours. Do not cover the bump, and do not get it wet. The test is positive if the area gets red and elevated. (See cough; respiratory problems, respiratory distress.)

Amniocentesis is a procedure that removes amniotic fluid from the amniotic sac for testing

X-ray. This can check the bones, including the extremities, the skull and spine, sinuses, neck, chest, and abdomen.

Chest x-rays show the lung, the heart, and the rib cage.

X-ray of the hands shows the child's bone age. That is important because the bone age correlates better with the child's bone maturation age than the chronologic age. In other words, a child's or adolescent's age does not tell us where his development stands, or if his height is normal or not, but the bone age does.

X-rays are also done with contrast materials. Those are substances that are used to enhance the examined structures. Upper gastrointestinal (UGI), barium swallow, barium enema, intravenous pyelography (IVP), and voiding cystourethrogram are these types of tests.

Upper GI: the child swallows some contrast material to check the esophagus, stomach, and part of the small bowel.

Barium swallow shows the mechanism of swallowing. A speech pathologist is often present to evaluate this test.

Barium enema means the introduction of a contrast material to the rectum to check the rectum and large bowels.

Intravenous pyelography (IVP): contrast material is injected to a vein, and the urinary system, including the kidneys, ureters, bladder, and urethra, are visualized.

Esophageal manometry is a test that measures the strength of the esophageal muscles as they push food to the stomach. It shows the work of the esophagus (esophagus is a tube connecting the throat to the stomach). This test checks for reflux and swallowing problems (dysphagia).

A small tube is placed into the child's nose, then down the throat into the esophagus.

Lung function tests (pulmonary function tests). These determine how well the lung works. The most common test is spirometry when the child blows into a tube connected to a machine called spirometer. It measures the rate of air flow and how much air the child's lung can hold.

Peak flow meter. This helps to evaluate the status of asthma at home. The child blows into a tube as hard as he can. The device measures how much air moves out of the lung with one strong exhalation. If it is decreased, that means the worsening of the asthma.

Voiding cystourethrogram (VCUG). This is an x-ray of the urinary tract. A contrast material is introduced with a tube (catheter) to the urethra, and when the urinary bladder is full and the urination starts, that is the time when the x-rays are done. This is the way to check for reflux, namely when some urine goes toward the kidneys instead of the whole amount of urine leaving the body through the urethra. (See urinary tract infection.)

Computed tomography (CAT scan or CT scan). CT scan is a series of x-ray images to look at structures inside of the body.

The most common are the head, abdominal, and chest CT scans. But all other structures of the body can be checked.

Young children need sedation (medicine to make the child sleepy) before the test.

Teenage girls need to let the doctor know if they might be pregnant before x-ray or CT scan.

CT urography. This is an examination of the kidneys, ureters, and bladder after intravenous contrast administration.

Sonography or ultrasonography. Sonography uses high frequency sound waves and produces images of internal organs.

Sonography is done without anesthesia, it is not painful, and there is no radiation.

Different organs can be checked:

- A baby's brain can be examined if the soft spot is open.
- Neck and the thyroid gland.
- Heart (heart sonogram is called echocardiogram or echo).
- The chest cavity.
- Abdomen including liver, spleen, and pancreas.
- Kidneys and bladder.
- Male and female genitals. To check the uterus, there is a so-called transvaginal ultrasound. A device is placed into the vagina.
- Bones, joints, and tissues can be checked as well.

Hearing test. The first hearing test is done in the newborn nursery. Hearing test for babies is done with a test called auditory brainstem evoked response (ABER). This test checks the response of brain waves to sounds.

Hearing test for children checks the child's response when hearing a sound.

Vision test. Vision test for babies is called visually evoked potential. This test checks the responses of the baby's brain waves to light.

Screening of vision for children vision charts are used.

Magnetic Resonance Imaging (MRI). This serves the same purpose as CT scan, but it uses magnetic fields instead of x-rays.

Some children need sedation before the test.

Nuclear scans. These use a small amount of radioactive materials and watch their accumulation in the targeted organ. Bone, thyroid, and kidney scans are often used.

Positron emission tomography (PET scan). This uses a radioactive drug to see how tissues and organs are functioning.

Electrocardiogram (ECG or EKG). This checks the electricity produced by the heart.

Echocardiogram (echo). This is a sonogram of the heart. It can provide information about the size, structure, and pumping capacity of the heart.

Electromyography (EMG). This evaluates the electrical activity produced by skeletal muscles.

Electroencephalography (EEG). This shows the electric activity of the brain.

Procedures, equipment

Catheterization. Catheterization is a procedure when a flexible tube (catheter) is placed into an organ.

Catheterization of different organs serves different purposes.

Cardiac catheterization is a procedure when a tube with a video camera is inserted to a blood vessel and moved to the heart to diagnose certain heart conditions.

Urinary catheterization is a procedure when a catheter is introduced to the urethra and moved to the urinary bladder. Urine is obtained from there and sent to the laboratory for urinalysis and culture (this is a sterile urine sample), to see if any bacteria is present.

After surgery, often a urinary catheter is placed to the bladder for a longer time to check the urine output (Foley catheter).

Endoscopy. Endoscope is a lighted flexible instrument that can see different hollow organs. Tissue samples also can be taken by the endoscope. This procedure is called biopsy. The sample obtained by the biopsy is examined under a microscope by a pathologist.

Arthroscopy. This is a procedure when a catheter is introduced to a joint to examine that joint.

Bronchoscopy. This is a procedure when the doctor, usually a pulmonologist, puts down a tube (bronchoscope) into the lung through the mouth.

Nebulizer. This is a machine that delivers medications in a form of aerosol.

Inhaler. This is a small device that delivers puffs from medications.

Aero Chamber. This is a tube that is attached to the inhaler. It channels the medication to the airways more effectively.

Upper endoscopy (esophagogastroduodenoscopy). The endoscope is introduced through the mouth, and it examines the esophagus, stomach, and part of the small bowels.

Colonoscopy. This is an endoscopy. The endoscope is introduced into the rectum and examines the rectum and large bowels.

Cystoscopy. This is an endoscopy when the endoscope is introduced into the urethra to check the urinary bladder.

Colposcopy. This is a procedure that examines female organs, the vulva, vagina, and cervix, with an endoscope.

Laryngoscopy. This is an endoscopy. A device called a laryngoscope is used by an ENT (ear, nose, and throat) doctor to examine the throat, voice box (larynx), and the vocal cords.
Laryngoscope is also used to intubate the patient (the anesthesiologist inserts a tube called endotracheal tube into the larynx) for anesthesia or in an emergency for resuscitation.

Rhinoscopy. This is the procedure for examining the inside of the nose.

Thoracoscopy. This is an endoscopy. A flexible tube with a video camera is inserted in the chest through a small incision. The surgeon can examine the lungs, the pleural cavity, and the chest cavity. He can also do biopsies and some surgical procedures. Thoracoscopy is used for diagnosing and treating different conditions in the chest.

Lumbar puncture or spinal tap. A needle is introduced into the spine to obtain a small amount of spinal fluid. The fluid is tested in the laboratory. Medications and dyes can also be injected to the spinal fluid this way.

Bone marrow aspiration. This is a procedure when a small amount of bone marrow is taken out through a needle. The sample goes to the laboratory. It shows whether the blood cells are normal and checks for leukemia (blood cancer).

Bladder tap. This is the introduction of a needle into the urinary bladder to get a urine sample. This urine is sterile, so besides urinalysis, it can be checked for culture to see if any bacteria is present.

Lithotripsy. This is a noninvasive procedure that uses high energy shock waves to break up kidney stones.

Dialysis. This is a process that takes over the role of failing kidneys. The kidneys filtrate the blood and produce urine. This way, toxins are removed, and fluids are replaced.

There are two kinds of dialysis. Hemodialysis is a procedure where blood is removed from the body and pumped through a special filter (hemodialysis filter) where it gets cleaned and returns to the body.

Peritoneal dialysis is a procedure where a sterile solution is infused to the abdomen and drained. This solution absorbs waste from the child's blood. Peritoneal dialysis can be done at home at night when the child is sleeping.

Elastic bandage. This is often used to treat muscle strain. It is important to check that the skin is not cold and blue, so the bandage is not too tight.

Splint. This is a device that immobilizes the broken bone until it heals or switched to a cast.

Orthopedic cast. This is a shell made from plaster or fiberglass. It is generally used to stabilize a broken bone until it heals.

Bone reposition. This is the process when a displaced bone is returned to the original position. It often requires surgery.

Pavlik harness. This is a device that keeps the hips in a good position, while the baby can still move her legs. It treats congenital hip dysplasia, when the head of the thigh bone is not fully in the joint socket (see flatfoot and other orthopedic conditions).

Photo therapy. This is a process where the baby is placed under a special blue light that breaks down the bilirubin. The baby's eyes are covered with a well-fitting eye patch all the time. Proper fluid intake is important.

Exchange blood transfusion is a procedure that removes a certain amount of blood of the patient and replaces it with donor blood to remove abnormal blood.

Venous access (intravenous or IV). This can be achieved by introducing a needle or catheter into the vein.

Blood samples can be obtained this way, and fluids, medications, even nutrition can be provided to the sick child. The so-called *central line* gives access to larger veins, like the jugular vein on the neck.

PICC line or peripherally inserted central catheter is a long catheter that is inserted through a vein of the child's arm or leg and guided into a large vein close to the heart (superior or inferior vena cava).

Venous cutdown. This is an emergency procedure to get venous access. The vein is surgically exposed, and a cannula (tube) is inserted into the vein.

Umbilical artery catheter (UAC). This is a plastic tube that is introduced into the navel (umbilical) artery of a newborn.

Umbilical venous catheter (UVC). The catheter is inserted into the umbilical vein of a newborn.

Both the umbilical artery and venous catheter give access to a blood vessel. They are easily available for getting blood samples and giving fluids and medications.

Nasogastric tube (NG tube). This is a plastic tube of different sizes that is inserted through the nose into the stomach.

Orogastric tube (OG tube). A plastic tube is inserted through the mouth into the stomach. It comes in different sizes as well. Both the NG and OG tubes can be used to get fluid and air out of the stomach. It can be used for feeding.

Surgeries

Gastrostomy. This is a surgical procedure. A gastrostomy or G-tube is placed into the stomach through the abdomen. It gives access to the stomach for supplemental feeding, hydration, or medications.

Tracheotomy or tracheostomy. This is a procedure when a hole is made through the front of the neck and into the windpipe (trachea). A tube is placed into the hole, and the patient breathes through that tube.

This is often an emergency procedure when the airway is blocked and the patient cannot breathe through the nose or mouth.

Pacemaker. This is a small device that is placed under the skin in the chest to help control heartbeats.

Thoracocentesis. This is the introduction of a needle to the pleural cavity. The pleura is a two-layered membrane that surrounds the lungs. The space between the two layers is the pleural cavity. If air, fluid, or blood accumulates in this space, that needs to be removed with thoracocentesis.

Pericardiocentesis. Pericardiocentesis is a procedure, when a cardiac surgeon insert a needle to the chest, and removes fluid from around the heart.

Video-assisted thoracoscopic surgery (VATS). This is a surgery done via thoracoscopy. Thoracoscopy is a procedure when a small camera is inserted into the chest through incisions. It is used for diagnosing and treating different conditions in the chest.

Thoracotomy. This is a surgery to open the chest.

Tonsillectomy. Removal of the tonsils. The tonsils are located on each side of the back of the throat.

Adenoidectomy. Removal of the adenoids. The adenoids are situated behind the nose.

The tonsils and the adenoids are so-called lymphatic tissues, and as such, they are part of the immune system that fights infections.

Often tonsillectomy and adenoidectomy are performed at the same time (see sore throat).

Nasal cauterization. This is a procedure that applies a chemical substance silver nitrate or an electric devise to slightly burn the enlarged blood vessels in the nose to stop recurrent nosebleeds. A local anesthetic is used before the procedure.

Ear tubes. These are tiny tubes that are inserted into the eardrums at both ears. It drains and prevents accumulation of fluids behind the eardrums.

Cochlear implant surgery is done to help the child with profound hearing loss in both ears.

Craniotomy. This is a surgery to open the skull.

Ventriculoperitoneal shunt (VP shunt). This is a tube that is surgically placed to connect the chamber (ventricle) of the brain to the abdomen.

That way, it drains the excess of cerebrospinal fluid from the brain to the abdomen and decreases the pressure on the brain. It is usually used if the child has hydrocephalus (see head: large, small, and misshapen).

Craniofacial surgeries. Cleft lip and palate surgery, reposition or reshape the skull, face, jaw, and craniosynostosis surgery (see head large, small, misshapen).

Eye surgery. This is usually done if the child has lazy eye (amblyopia), and correction was not achieved by conservative therapy with eye patches or glasses.

Heart surgery. This is done if the child has significant congenital heart disease.

Appendectomy. Removal of the inflamed appendix. Appendix is a pouch-like sac of the large bowel, located on the right side of the abdomen (see stomachache).

Laparoscopy. This is a surgical procedure of the abdomen. Small incisions are made, and a camera is used to make diagnosis or surgery.

Hernia surgery. Repair can be done with laparoscopy.

Laparotomy. This is a surgical procedure. A large incision is made through the abdominal wall to have access into the abdominal cavity.

Nissen fundoplication. This is a surgical procedure to resolve severe gastroesophageal reflux disease (GERD).

Orchiopexy. This is a surgical procedure to bring down undescended testicles to the scrotum.

Circumcision. This is the surgical removal of the foreskin of the penis. It is done for ritual, traditional, or health reasons (see circumcision).

Organ transplantation. This is a medical procedure in which an organ is removed from the body of the donor and placed in the body of the recipient to replace a failing organ.

Orthopedic surgeries. Orthopedic surgeries treat conditions that affect the bones, tendons, joints, and muscles.

Hand surgery. Hand surgery treats children with congenital deformities and injuries of the hands and arms.

Dental procedures

Filling of cavities. This is the most common dental procedure.

Root canal procedure. This treats the pulp of the tooth, which is soft tissue inside of the tooth that contains nerves and vessels.

Tooth repatriation. This is the dental procedure that puts back the tooth that was broken off. Time is essential (see teething, tooth and gum problems).

Dental braces. These are devices used in orthodontics to align and straighten teeth.

Dental retainer. This is a device that keeps the teeth in place after the braces have been removed by the orthodontist.

Physicians, specialists, and subspecialists

Many specialties have doctors who only work with children, like neonatologists, pediatric ophthalmologist, pediatric cardiologists, pediatric endocrinologists, pediatric gastroenterologists, pediatric nephrologist, pediatric dermatologist, pediatric hematologists, pediatric gynecologists, pediatric neurologists, pediatric otolaryngologists, pediatric allergist/immunologists, pediatric pulmonologists, pediatric surgeons, pediatric intensivists, pediatric emergency medicine specialist, pediatric infectious disease specialists, pediatric geneticist, pediatric metabolic specialist, developmental-behavioral pediatrician, and adolescent medicine specialist.

Allergist is a specialist who treats allergies like hay fever and asthma.

Anesthesiologist is a medical doctor who administers anesthetics during surgery so the patient sleeps and has no pain. He monitors the patient all the time. Anesthesiologists also do pain medicine.

Cardiologist is a heart doctor who treats diseases and conditions of the heart and the circulatory system (blood vessels).

Dermatologist is a skin doctor.

Endocrinologist is a medical doctor who deals with glands and the hormones they make.

ENT doctor or otolaryngologist is a medical doctor whose field is the ear, nose, throat, and related structures of the head and neck.

Otologist or neurotologist is a subspecialist of otolaryngology who provides medical and surgical treatment of the inner ear and auditory nerve. Cochlear implant surgery is done by otologists.

Family physician is a medical doctor who takes care of people of all ages.

Gastroenterologist (GI doctor) is concerned with the digestive system, from the esophagus to the rectum.

Geneticist is a medical doctor who works with hereditary and genetic disorders.

Gynecologist (see obstetrician-gynecologist) is a medical doctor who deals with the health maintenance and the diseases of women.

Hematologist is a medical doctor who works with diseases and disorders of the blood.

Immunologist is a medical doctor whose concern is the immune system.

Infectious disease specialist is a medical doctor who diagnoses and treats infectious diseases.

A tropical medicine doctor is a doctor who specialized in the diagnosis, treatment, and prevention of diseases that are most common in the tropical climate.

Intensivist is a medical doctor who is specialized in the care of critically ill patients, usually in the intensive care unit (ICU).

Internist is a medical doctor who takes care of the health needs of adults.

Metabolic specialist is a medical doctor who works with metabolic diseases, the defects of the body's chemistry. He evaluates children who are suspected to have a metabolic disease.

Neonatologist is a medical doctor who takes care of premature and sick newborns, usually in the neonatal intensive care unit (NICU).

Nephrologist is a kidney specialist.

Neurologist is a medical doctor who deals with the nervous system.

Obstetrician-gynecologist (OB-GYN) is a medical doctor who takes care of women, including pregnancy and childbirth.

Oncologist is a medical doctor who deals with different kinds of cancers.

Ophthalmologist is an eye doctor.

Orthopedic surgeon is a medical doctor who treats problems of the bone, joints, ligaments, and the muscles.

Pathologist is a medical doctor who examines bodies, body tissues, and performs laboratory tests to help to make the diagnosis of different medical conditions.

Pediatrician is a medical doctor who deals with the health maintenance and diseases of infants, children, and adolescents.

Adolescent medicine specialist provides care for adolescents and young adults.

Physiatrist is a medical doctor whose specialty is physical medicine and rehabilitation (PM&R).

Psychiatrist is a medical doctor who is specialized to diagnose and treat mental disorders.

Developmental pediatrician makes the diagnosis, and treats disorders of development, learning, and behavior.

Pulmonologist is a doctor whose specialty is to treat lung diseases, including asthma.

Radiologist is a medical doctor who is specialized in diagnosing medical conditions, diseases, and injuries using medical imaging techniques. These are x-rays, computed tomography (CAT scan or CT scan), magnetic resonance imaging (MRI), nucleic scans, positron emission tomography (PET scan), and sonography (ultrasound). Some radiologists also treat patients, like interventional radiologists and radiation oncologists.

Rheumatologist is a medical doctor who treats disorders of the joints, ligaments, and muscles.

Sleep doctor is specialized to diagnose and treat sleep disturbances and disorders.

Sports medicine doctor deals with physical fitness and the prevention and treatment of sports injuries.

Urologist is a medical doctor whose focus is the urinary tract and the male reproductive organs.

Surgeons

Cardiac surgeon is a medical doctor who performs surgeries of the heart and great vessels.

Cardiovascular surgeon operates on the heart and blood vessels.

Cardiothoracic surgeon is specialized to do surgeries inside the chest cavity, treating conditions of the heart, lungs, and other organs.

Thoracic surgeon is a medical doctor who deals with surgical diseases of the chest.

Colorectal surgeon is a medical doctor who specialized in the surgical treatment of the lower digestive tract, the large intestine, and the rectum.

Craniofacial surgeon is a medical doctor who treats children with deformities of the head, skull, face, jaw, neck, and related structures.

General surgeon is a physician who takes care of patients with surgical conditions, from diagnosis and surgery to postoperative management.

Hand surgeon is a medical doctor who specializes in the treatment of the hand, wrist, and forearm.

Neurosurgeon is a medical doctor who deals with surgical conditions of the nervous system and associated structures.

Pediatric surgeon is the general surgeon of children.

Plastic surgeon is a medical doctor who works on restoration, reconstruction, and alteration of the human body.

It includes craniofacial surgeries and hand surgeries (see above).

Clinical professional doctors

Audiologist is a health-care professional who evaluates hearing loss and related disorders and gives recommendations for their improvement.

Optometrist is a doctor of optometry who is primarily dealing with the diagnosis and treatment of vision changes, including prescribing and distributing eyeglasses.

Podiatrist is a doctor of podiatric medicine who treats disorders of the foot and ankle.

Psychologist is a mental health professional who has a graduate degree in psychology. A psychologist evaluates and treats behavior and mental processes.

Other health professionals

Anesthetist is a certified registered nurse anesthetist (CRNA) who administers certain drugs to have patients sleep during surgery, working under the supervision of an anesthesiologist.

Dietician is a health-care professional who helps to regulate the patient's diet according to the medical needs.

Medical assistant is a health professional who supports the work of physicians.

Nurses are professionals who help doctors to take care of patients.

Nurse practitioners (NP) are advanced practice registered nurses. They can diagnose diseases and treat patients.

Occupational therapist (OT) is a professional who helps children and adults to improve their capability to function.

Optician is a technician who designs and fits lenses and glass frames.

Physical therapist or physiotherapist (PT) helps to promote mobility and function through exercises and other means.

Physician assistant is a professional who works under the supervision of a doctor. He goes to the patient first before the doctor.

Respiratory therapist is a professional who gives respiratory treatments to patients ordered by the doctor.

Social worker is a professional who helps to solve problems for the sick and disadvantaged.

Speech therapist or speech and language therapist is a professional who evaluates and treats speech and language problems and voice and swallowing disorders.

Surgical technician is a professional who prepares the equipment for surgery.

Doctors of dental care

Dentist is a doctor whose field is the teeth and the oral cavity.

Endodontist is a doctor who does root canal procedures.

Oral surgeon is a doctor who performs surgeries of the oral cavity and jaw.

Orthodontist is a doctor dealing with the correction of irregular teeth.

Periodontist is a dentist who specializes in the prevention, diagnosis, and treatment of gum diseases.

Pediatric dentists are specialized to treat children.

Index